Creation Ethics

Creation Ethics

Reproduction, Genetics, and Quality of Life

DAVID DeGRAZIA

OXFORD
UNIVERSITY PRESS

OXFORD
UNIVERSITY PRESS

Oxford University Press, Inc., publishes works that further
Oxford University's objective of excellence
in research, scholarship, and education.

Oxford   New York
Auckland   Cape Town   Dar es Salaam   Hong Kong   Karachi
Kuala Lumpur   Madrid   Melbourne   Mexico City   Nairobi
New Delhi   Shanghai   Taipei   Toronto

With offices in
Argentina   Austria   Brazil   Chile   Czech Republic   France   Greece
Guatemala   Hungary   Italy   Japan   Poland   Portugal   Singapore
South Korea   Switzerland   Thailand   Turkey   Ukraine   Vietnam

Copyright © 2012 Oxford University Press

Published by Oxford University Press, Inc.
198 Madison Avenue, New York, New York 10016

www.oup.com

Oxford is a registered trademark of Oxford University Press

Library of Congress Cataloging-in-Publication Data
DeGrazia, David.
Creation ethics : reproduction, genetics, and quality of life / David DeGrazia.
    p.   cm.
ISBN 978-0-19-538963-0 (alk. paper)
1. Human reproductive technology—Moral and ethical aspects.
2. Medical genetics—Moral and ethical aspects. I. Title.
RG133.5.D456   2012
174.2'96042—dc23   2011035709

9 8 7 6 5 4 3 2 1

Printed in the United States of America
on acid-free paper

CONTENTS

Creation Ethics

1

Introduction

To create is to bring into existence. Creation may involve simply making something, or it may involve invention—coming up with something new. Human beings create myriad things: buildings and books, thermometers and theories, microphones and marriages, paintings and peace treaties. Human beings even create, or decide not to create, human beings.

First, and most obviously, we human beings create other human beings through *procreation*—reproduction, as it is usually called. Most human reproduction occurs naturally, by way of sexual intercourse. Some reproduction, though, is made possible by artificial means such as in vitro fertilization. And, of course, people sometimes decide to terminate the process of reproductive creation by aborting pregnancies.

In addition to creating new human beings, people sometimes deliberately create, or refrain from creating, particular *kinds* of human beings—that is, human beings with *particular characteristics*—by controlling reproduction in various ways: carefully choosing a reproductive partner, or a sperm or egg donor; deciding to carry a fetus to term or aborting in view of what they think the offspring will or would be like; employing prenatal genetic diagnosis and selecting embryos on the basis of test results. At some point in the future, we will probably have the options of prenatal genetic therapy and prenatal genetic enhancement, which will extend the power to create human beings with particular characteristics.

Sometimes human creative activity is self-directed because people sometimes engage in *self-creation*. Although a person does not literally bring herself into existence, she may work to change certain of her traits or acquire new traits in an effort to become a different sort of person. Deliberate self-improvement is nothing new, but novel technologies expand the tools available for such projects. Genetic enhancements are likely to be added to the toolbox of self-creation.

Finally, our reproductive acts, considered collectively, create *new generations*. Importantly for future generations, our choices determine not only who will come into being, but also what sort of world future generations will inherit. Thus, we not only create future generations but, in a sense, we create the state of the world in which they will find themselves.

The choices we make about creating other human beings, particular kinds of human beings, ourselves, and future generations—not to mention their world— all provoke ethical and philosophical issues. Many of these issues involve reproduction, genetics, or both. The term *reprogenetics* is sometimes used to refer to the intersection of the fields of assisted reproduction, human genetics, and embryo research. Some portions of this book will concern ethical and philosophical issues in reprogenetics, thus understood. But the scope of this book is considerably broader insofar as it also addresses ethical and philosophical issues connected with reproductive choices, considered independently of genetics, and ethical and philosophical issues pertaining to genetics, considered independently of reproduction. Moreover, in thinking about future generations, we will explore ethical and philosophical issues less in relation to reproduction than in relation to how our lifestyles affect the world that later people will inherit, with foreseeable effects on their quality of life.

In characterizing the topics to be explored in this book, I have several times made reference to ethical and philosophical issues. It bears mentioning that the discussion of distinctively philosophical issues—such as "At what point in the reproductive process does one of us come into being?," "What is human nature?," and "Do future people have interests?"—will primarily be in the service of ethics. That is, we address the philosophical issue in order to achieve sufficient conceptual or metaphysical clarity to put us in a good position to address the ethical issues. This is not at all to deny the independent importance and interest of the philosophical issues (which fascinate me); it is simply to make explicit that this book is primarily a work in ethics. *The overarching aim of this book is to illuminate a cluster of ethical issues connected to human reproduction and human genetics through the lens of moral philosophy.*

RELATIONSHIP TO EXISTING LITERATURE

The ethical issues addressed in the present volume are represented by a vast literature. This literature comprises many books and an enormous number of articles. The book-length discussions include such monographs as Heyd's

Genethics, Steinbock's *Life Before Birth*, Kamm's *Creation and Abortion*, Silver's *Remaking Eden*, Glover's *Choosing Children*, Green's *Babies by Design*, Harris' *Enhancing Evolution*, and Buchanan's *Beyond Humanity?*; they also include such anthologies as Savulescu and Bostrom's *Human Enhancement* and Roberts and Wasserman's *Harming Future Persons*.[1] These are just some of the better books on the topics explored here. How will my book add to this impressive literature? How is it distinctive?

As suggested by their titles, each of the representative books just mentioned focuses more narrowly than *Creation Ethics*, which covers an exceptionally wide range of topics. Sometimes, of course, breadth of coverage comes at the cost of superficiality. I believe, however, that within the literature on ethical issues in reproduction and genetics, *Creation Ethics* offers a unique combination of breadth and philosophical depth. If I have succeeded in my aims, another un-usual feature is the simultaneous achievement of accessibility, on the one hand, and precision and argumentative rigor, on the other. The book is also well versed and up-to-date in ethical and philosophical theory while being scientifically well informed wherever science is crucial to the discussion. Needless to say, many discussions feature one of these two academic virtues in the absence of the other.

Creation Ethics is also somewhat unusual in addressing reproductive ethics without shying away from prenatal moral status and the attendant ethical issues of abortion and embryo research. In confronting these issues, Chapter 2 strives to avoid the one-sidedness that characterizes so much work in this area. Indeed, among discussions that arrive at a definite position, perhaps none is fairer to the vision and arguments that animate the opposing side. I take some pride in believing that the book as a whole is exceptional in the degree to which it takes alternative moral visions seriously.

Several, more specific distinguishing features of *Creation Ethics* will become apparent in the overview of the six major chapters.

OVERVIEW

Chapter 2, "Prenatal Moral Status and Ethics," is the book's longest chapter. Its first major task is to defend a framework for understanding prenatal moral status. The framework has three key components: (1) an account of the essence, numerical identity, and origins of human beings; (2) a view about the relevance of sentience to moral status; and (3) a version of the "time-relative interest ac-count" (TRIA) of the harm of death and its relevance to prenatal moral status.

According to the first component, we are essentially human animals or or-ganisms so that our origins—the point in the reproductive process when we come into being—and the criteria for our numerical identity—that is, for our continuing to exist over time—are to be understood in biological terms. This view, which I defended in *Human Identity and Bioethics* and which has been most comprehensively defended by Eric Olson[2], swims against analytical philosophy's mainstream currents, which carry various psychological views of our essence, origins, and identity. The biological view suggests that we come into existence as early as conception and no later than two weeks after conception, when integration among the embryo's cells has been unambiguously achieved and spontaneous twinning is no longer possible. I argue that we come into existence between several days and two weeks after conception, but acknowledge that the conception view is defensible.

The second component of the tripartite framework claims a strong connection between sentience and moral status. Sentience is sufficient for having interests and therefore, I argue, for moral status. Unlike most liberals who embrace similar views, though, I do not assume that sentience is *necessary* for interests and moral status. Indeed, I argue that the view that *potential* for sentience and/or personhood is sufficient for moral status is about as compelling as the view that sentience is necessary. Thus, for all I have argued so far, a coherent pro-life view remains standing. For, once one of us comes into being at or shortly after conception, that being possesses the relevant potential. One aim of this discussion is to clarify appeals to potential, which are routinely misrepresented by liberal critics.

While the first two components of the tripartite framework leave the argumentative door open to pro-life views, the third closes the door by deploying a version of the TRIA of the harm of death. Developed by Jeff McMahan, the TRIA holds that an evaluation of the harm of death must take into account not only (1) the value of the future life lost by the individual who dies, but also (2) the degree of psychological relatedness between the individual just before dying and the later individual who otherwise would have lived.[3] Whereas McMahan develops the TRIA such that the presentient fetus has no interests and no moral status—indeed, on his psychological view of our essence, identity, and origins, the presentient fetus and later sentient fetus are *numerically distinct individuals*—I consider an alternative understanding according to which a presentient fetus has significantly diminished (but not the absence of) interests and moral status. This more moderate position can be defended on the basis of (1) the presentient fetus' numerical identity to a possible future individual like us (a type of potential), grounding its moral status, and (2) the absence of mental life, which justifies the claim of *relatively weak* time-relative interests and moral status. My tripartite framework ultimately supports a liberal position on prenatal moral status and, consequently, on the ethics of abortion and embryo research insofar as the killing of fetuses and embryos is judged to be considerably less morally problematic than the killing of sentient beings and persons, if problematic at all.

But is my framework justified? It is one thing to provide a framework a preliminary defense, but quite another to show that the strongest possible objections cannot overturn it. The strongest opposition to a liberal position like mine is found in the literature on the ethics of abortion, so the discussion turns to what I take to be the three strongest arguments represented in that literature: the Future-Like-Ours Argument, the Appeal to the Practical Necessity of Early Moral Protection, and the Appeal to Our Essence and Kind Membership. After rebutting these arguments, thereby strengthening the case for my framework, I turn to what many philosophers consider the strongest argument for a pro-choice view: the Good Samaritan Argument (GSA). I contend that the success of the GSA is highly uncertain. So the TRIA remains crucial to my defense of a liberal position.

Perhaps surprisingly, I next argue that there are respectable grounds for doubting the liberal position I have defended. For example, I might be mistaken about the defensibility of the TRIA. Or, even if I'm right that my framework, including the TRIA, and the liberal position it supports comprise a reasonable position, perhaps the strongest pro-life position is about equally reasonable. Thus, I argue, there remains room for reasonable disagreement about our origins and prenatal moral status, as well as their ethical implications. In response to such ontological-moral pluralism, or plurality of reasonable views, I shift the discussion from moral philosophy to political philosophy.

From the standpoint of political philosophy, I argue, justified public policies regarding abortion and embryo research must be fairly liberal. In defense of this thesis, I highlight the three pivotal assumptions on which the pro-life position rests: (1) We human beings come into existence at conception; (2) We have full moral status—including a right to life—throughout our existence; and (3) If we have full moral status from the time of conception, then abortion and embryo research are impermissible (with few, if any, exceptions). *The pro-life view requires all three of these controversial assumptions.* Yet, by this point in the discussion, we have found that each can reasonably be doubted. I argue that the government must not impose significant restrictions on the liberty of pregnant women and biomedical researchers on the basis of such contestable assumptions. This supports broadly liberal policies.

The last major section provides details. The analysis vindicates most of the legal status quo regarding abortion in the United States, including the prohibition of public funds for this procedure, but it rejects the Supreme Court's ruling on "partial-birth" abortions. My analysis also carves out a "no responsibility" exception (which includes but is not limited to rape) to the prohibition of public funds. In the analysis of embryo research policy, which gives special attention to embryonic stem-cell research, one notable result is my rejection of the view that it is permissible to use spare embryos from fertility clinics *but not to create embryos for research purposes*. Both, I argue, are permissible—unless and until research demonstrates that use of "adult" stem cells has benefits comparable to those afforded by use of embryonic stem cells.

Chapter 3, "Creation Through Genetic Enhancement," addresses self-creation (self-shaping or -transformation) and the creation of particular sorts of human beings—that is, human beings with desired characteristics—by way of genetic enhancement. Rather than providing a comprehensive analysis of the ethics of genetic enhancement, which would require several chapters if not an entire book, the ethical analysis is focused through the conceptual lenses of human identity and human nature. The first section explores the concept of enhancement and finds two conceptions—one that contrasts enhancement with treatment, another that understands enhancement in terms of expanding capacities—about equally defensible and useful. The next section presents examples of possible genetic enhancements of the future. Eight have a fairly clear basis in current scientific understanding and are, in that sense, relatively near-term. Two further examples have the feel of science fiction, given the current state of technology, yet are entirely conceivable. One of these thought-experiments involves the gradual evolution via genetic enhancement of *post-humans*, a new hominid species that is greatly superior to *Homo sapiens* in various respects. The second thought-experiment features *post-persons*, who are characterized by their superior moral agency. In view of their vastly superior moral capacities, post-persons entertain a new ontological distinction between reliable moral agents (them) and haphazard moral agents (us). Post-persons wonder whether they have higher moral status than persons, just as persons have traditionally regarded themselves as having higher moral status than nonhuman animals.

With this background, the chapter proceeds to the primary philosophical and ethical issues. First, since many concerns about enhancements are expressed in the language of identity, what is the relationship between biomedical enhancement and identity? I argue that here it is absolutely crucial to distinguish between *numerical identity*—the relation something has to itself in being one and the same thing over time—and *narrative identity*, which concerns a particular person's self-conception.[4] It becomes apparent that the only enhancements, genetic or otherwise, that anyone is ever likely to use would not disrupt numerical identity—that is, eliminate one individual and replace her with another—but would at most change a person's narrative identity. But, then, what's wrong with that? The most promising answer appeals to authenticity, so this concept is analyzed. Ultimately, the appeal to authenticity is found unpersuasive as an objection to genetic or any other kind of enhancement.

The chapter proceeds to objections that appeal to perceived risks to human nature—and, in some variations of the objections, to humanity itself. In addressing the concern about human nature, I present the structure of the underlying reasoning and evaluate each step. First, it is assumed that there is such a thing as human nature. I briefly defend this assumption. Second, it is assumed that genetic enhancement threatens human nature. After exploring what it would mean to threaten human nature, I argue that the nearer-term possibilities of genetic enhancement considered earlier would not pose such a threat whereas the emergence of post-humans or post-persons would. The third premise is that threatening human nature is morally unacceptable. In response, I first argue that there is nothing *inherently* wrong with threatening—that is, surpassing or changing—human nature. But consequentialist concerns about risks to humanity (not to human nature itself) prove more significant: The emergence of post-humans or post-persons could endanger humanity due to a massive power differential between humans and the superior beings. Unenhanced human beings, that is, might be vulnerable to exploitation, domination, or worse.

Considering the possibility of such a disastrous outcome, what sort of precautions would be appropriate? I argue that prohibiting genetic enhancement in order to foreclose the possibility of disaster would be no more sensible than it would have been to prohibit travel by ships and airplanes in view of the possibility of lethal epidemics or annihilation through warfare. I proceed to more moderate strategies for reducing the long-term risks of genetic enhancement while protecting possible benefits from this technology, and ultimately defend the view I call Moderate Regulation.

Chapter 4, "Prenatal Genetic Interventions," tightly integrates the themes of reproduction and genetics as it addresses three types of interventions: (1) prenatal genetic diagnosis (PGD), the testing of gametes (sperm or egg cells) prior to fertilization, embryos prior to implantation, or fetuses in utero; (2) prenatal genetic therapy (PGT), genetic therapy performed on a gamete, embryo, or fetus; and (3) prenatal genetic enhancement (PGE), the genetic enhancement of a gamete, embryo, or fetus. PGD is a current reality, with an ever-expanding range of conditions for which testing is possible. PGT and PGE are both fairly likely to become available in the not-so-distant future. Even if PGE is not officially permitted when PGT is, the blurred boundary between therapy and enhancement will probably permit PGE to sneak in under the guise of therapy.

The chapter begins with an overview of the current state of reprogenetics. The next section, the chapter's longest, addresses three prominent objections to prenatal genetic diagnosis that have been advanced by disability advocates: (1) the loss-of-support argument, (2) the "expressivist objection," and (3) the thesis that disabilities are really just differences. Although commonly voiced, the loss-of-support argument proves easy to rebut. The other two objections to PGD, however, demand detailed investigations. The expressivist objection argues that

PGD conveys hurtful messages regarding persons who have the disabilities for which PGD tests, thereby wronging those persons. I argue that, when directed at prospective parents who use PGD, the objection misfires because parents do not necessarily express the negative messages attributed in the objection; when the objection targets routine, aggressive promotion of PGD by medical institutions, though, it is more persuasive. According to the third objection to PGD considered here, disabilities are not objectively disadvantageous conditions, but rather different ways of functioning that prove disadvantageous only as a result of contingent social conditions. Responding to this objection requires an excursion into value theory, which features competing accounts of what ultimately constitutes human well-being. Against recent trends, I defend a qualified subjective account of well-being. From this perspective, I contend that disabilities are not *necessarily* injurious to an individual's overall well-being, but they typically impose disadvantages (even when social accommodations are abundant) that it is not unreasonable to want to avoid in one's offspring. PGD, I conclude, is a legitimate means of pursuing this parental aim.

The next major section takes up prenatal genetic therapy. It seems natural to think that, if a given PGT appears sufficiently safe and offers a better benefit-risk ratio than any alternative, it is justified. Several commentators, however, have worried that changing an individual's genome would change essential properties, thereby creating a numerically distinct individual—which would hardly be therapeutic to the original individual! Thus, these commentators question the legitimacy of PGT (and PGE). Partly in response to this line of reasoning, I defend a *Robustness Thesis*: Once we come into existence, our numerical identity is robust in the sense of being likely to survive any genetic interventions we might realistically expect in the name of therapy or enhancement. On my view, as explained in Chapter 2, we are essentially human animals or organisms so that the criteria for our continued existence over time are biological. But a human organism can undergo all sorts of genetic changes, whether intentionally produced or accidentally incurred, without going out of existence. If a genetic change had caused the prenatal being I once was to grow into a blond person, or someone with more musical talent, that would have changed my life and self-story in certain ways, but *I* would have been the one to live that life; these changes would not have killed or eliminated the organism. Since changes of narrative identity are not inherently problematic, intentional changes of a given individual's genome are not inherently problematic—at least for any reason related to identity. But the Robustness Thesis concerns identity after someone comes into being. Before someone comes into existence, changes to her precursor genetic materials may result in a numerically distinct individual's coming to be. I argue, however, that this metaphysical fact in no way casts doubt on the moral appropriateness of PGT performed on gametes or (if we come into existence shortly after conception) on the early embryo. I also contend, against the bioethics mainstream, that germline PGT—whose effects are heritable by later generations—is, in general, no less justified than somatic-cell PGT, whose effects are limited to the recipient of therapy.

Prenatal genetic enhancement raises some unique issues, which are taken up in the final major section of Chapter 4. First, can PGE be in the best interests of the child-to-be? In answering affirmatively, I contend that we should understand the best-interests standard as protecting a child's *essential* interests, explain how PGE can be sufficiently safe to attempt responsibly, and argue that PGE need not violate a child's "right to an open future." Second, does a decision to use PGE express morally objectionable parental attitudes? Does such use display insufficient regard for the "giftedness" of children? I argue that it does not. Finally, I take up residual concerns about possible social effects of PGE. Some of these concerns are sufficiently serious that I recommend a few restrictions on PGE.

Chapter 5, "Bearing Children in Wrongful Life Cases," opens with descriptions of two devastating genetic conditions: Tay-Sachs disease and Lesch-Nyham syndrome. These conditions are plausibly regarded as making the lives of those who have them not worth living. It is commonly asserted that knowingly or negligently to bring a child into the world with such a condition wrongs the child—hence the concept of *wrongful life*. Standard analyses of wrongful life incorporate the idea that bearing a child in such a case *harms* her. Yet our ordinary understanding of harm is comparative: A harms B only if A makes B *worse off* than B (1) *was before* the intervention claimed to be harmful or (2) *would have been* had the intervention not occurred. But neither of these two types of comparison seems possible in the present sort of case: Before an individual is brought into existence, she *was not*; and had she not been brought into existence, she *would not have been*. So how can she have been made worse off by being brought into existence?

This puzzle motivates the chapter's first line of inquiry: Does it ever wrong someone to bring him into existence and, if so, how can we coherently explain the nature of the wrong? After briefly reviewing strategies for making sense of the charge of wrongful life, including some that hold that the child brought into being is wronged without being harmed, I argue that at least one of these strategies is successful. There are wrongful life cases: cases in which someone is wronged by being brought into existence.

Certain facts about procreation motivate a more radical question than the one just answered. All human life involves harms. So to bring someone into existence is to guarantee that she will be harmed. Of course, nearly all lives also include benefits, which might be thought to compensate for the harms in many or most cases. But no one who is brought into existence consents in advance to the package of benefits and harms that her life will contain. And it seems plausible to judge that it is wrong to impose harm on someone, without her consent, in order to afford her "pure benefits" (benefits that do not involve the removal or prevention of harm). This motivates the radical question: Might every instance of procreation be wrong, and, if not, what can justify the unconsented imposition of harm? Because David Benatar and Seanna Shiffrin have presented the most developed arguments for a thoroughly anti-procreation position,[5] I examine and respond to their arguments in detail.

This discussion leads me to the following claims: (1) In paradigm wrongful life cases—in which the life would not be worth living—procreation is wrong; (2) In other cases involving the predictable imposition of a disability or life circumstance that is severe but not so bad as to make life not worth living, procreation is (strongly) pro tanto wrong; and (3) In those cases involving only exposure to the ordinary harms of human life, procreation is (weakly) pro tanto wrong. These claims provoke the question of what considerations might justify procreating in view of its (weak or strong) pro tanto wrongness. My reply invokes the value of procreative freedom as well as a consideration that I call the "undeluded gladness factor." The latter is connected to the thesis that those who are glad to be alive are generally not to be second-guessed about their belief that their lives are worth living, a belief that underscores the point that life involves not only burdens but opportunities. The chapter closes by setting up Chapter 6 with this question: In deciding whether to have children, what criteria should prospective parents use? In short, what do all parents owe their children?

Chapter 6, "Bearing and Caring for Children with Disadvantage," tackles this and other questions. The chapter focuses on procreation with the intention of *raising* the created child rather than giving her up for adoption (although some of the discussion also bears on the ethics of adoption). The disadvantages at issue include both substantial disabilities and predictable, obstacle-posing life circumstances such as entrenched poverty and slavery.

The first section examines our intuitive reactions to a wide variety of hypothetical cases as a method for identifying a defensible standard for "procreation plus parenting." The analysis leads to a standard according to which parents owe their children the following: (1) lives worth living (2) in which their basic needs—essential interests—are reasonably expected to be met (some exceptions being tolerable where failure to meet basic needs is due to circumstances beyond the parents' control), and (3) doing more for them where parents can without undue sacrifice. This standard is accompanied by a detailed list of children's basic needs, but whether freedom from avoidable disability belongs on that list is left an open question. The remainder of the chapter addresses the ethics of procreating from the standpoint of different types of procreative choice.

It is argued in the next section that in *same-individual choices*—choices between having a child with a major disadvantage and having the same child without the disadvantage—the importance of procreative freedom is straightforwardly outweighed by the child's interests. In the section that follows, I argue that procreative freedom carries greater weight with *different-number choices*: choices between having a child with disadvantage versus not having a child. Turning next to *same-number choices*—where parents can have a child with disadvantage or, by delaying conception or aborting and conceiving again, have a different child free of the disadvantage—we encounter the *nonidentity problem*, which generates several paradoxes about ethics and about which a massive literature has grown.[6] A variety of strategies for resolving the nonidentity problem are laid out—perhaps more lucidly and accessibly than one can find elsewhere in the literature—and appraised, and a solution is suggested. The chapter's final section sketches a view of "wrongful disadvantage" and draws implications for the ethics of procreating in a variety of circumstances in which prospective parents may find or place themselves. The discussion takes up very young parents, single parents, gay or lesbian parents, elderly parents, indigent parents, uninvolved "yuppie" and/or narcissistic parents, and those who would use reproductive cloning as a means to becoming parents.

The book concludes with Chapter 7, "Obligations to Future Generations," which opens with the question of what we, who are now contributing to global climate change, owe to future generations, who will inherit its harmful effects. This brings us to the central topic of the chapter. Collectively, the procreative acts of a given generation create a new generation; and, of course, the new generation will go on to create another generation, and so on for as long as humanity exists. Moreover, any given generation creates, or at least greatly affects, the conditions of the world that later generations will inherit. Because our choices so greatly affect the quality of life of future generations, it may seem obvious that we have moral obligations concerning our effects on the world that we leave our descendants. But our moral obligations apply most straightforwardly in dealings with contemporaries. Difficult philosophical issues confront the thesis that we have obligations to those who will exist only in the future.

The chapter is organized into sections that address distinct questions. First, do future persons have interests, moral status, and rights? Can we have obligations *to* them and not just *regarding* them? I answer the second question affirmatively on the basis of the fact that future persons *will* have interests, moral status, and rights. In doing so, I expose and rebut what I call *the temporally-bound correlativity thesis*, which holds that one can have obligations to particular individuals at a given time if and only if they have rights against one at that same time.

Second, are our obligations to future generations a matter of justice? A negative answer is supported by a classical view of the circumstances of justice. Rooted historically in the contract tradition of ethics, this view maintains that justice can obtain only among parties that are roughly equal in power and capable of reciprocity. I contest the classical view and argue that what we owe future generations is a matter of justice. I also show how the contract theories of Rawls and Scanlon can be plausibly extended in ways that support my claim.

Third, even if future persons have full moral status, and our obligations to them are a matter of justice, should their interests nevertheless count less than ours because of their temporal distance from us? Identifying and rebutting several leading arguments that favor the discounting of future persons' interests, I reject any type of systematic discounting.

Fourth, in view of nonidentity, how can we explain the wrong of irresponsible policy choices and individual decisions that leave a compromised world for future generations? The nonidentity problem arises in connection with future generations because different choices—say, addressing energy needs with solar power versus addressing them with nuclear power whose waste products cannot be safely disposed of for more than a few generations—will lead, eventually, to the existence of different individuals. A decision may predictably and irresponsibly result in a lower quality of life for individuals who exist several generations later but, unless their lives are not worth living, it is difficult to explain why the decision is wrong. My solution includes a novel suggestion for uniting the deontological approach of "what we owe to each other" and an impersonal, consequentialist approach to ethics.

If this book achieves its purpose, it will illuminate each of the topics connected with human reproduction and/or human genetics that are addressed herein: prenatal moral status and the ethics of abortion and embryo research; the ethics of genetic enhancement as it relates to human identity and human nature; the ethics of prenatal genetic diagnosis, therapy, and enhancement; wrongful life and the prerogative to have children; more broadly, the ethics of procreating with the intention of parenting; and obligations to future generations.

NOTES

1. See David Heyd, *Genethics* (Berkeley: University of California Press, 1992); Bonnie Steinbock, *Life Before Birth* (New York: Oxford University Press, 1992); Frances Kamm, *Creation and Abortion* (New York: Oxford University Press, 1992); Lee Silver, *Remaking Eden* (New York: Avon, 1997); Jonathan Glover, *Choosing Children* (Oxford: Clarendon, 2006); Ronald Green, *Babies by Design* (New Haven, CT: Yale University Press, 2007); John Harris, *Enhancing Evolution* (Princeton: Princeton University Press, 2007); Allen Buchanan, *Beyond*

Humanity? (New York: Oxford University Press, 2011); Julian Savulescu and Nick Bostrom (eds.), *Human Enhancement* (Oxford: Oxford University Press, 2009); and Melinda Roberts and David Wasserman (eds.), *Harming Future Persons* (Dordrecht, Netherlands: Springer, 2009).

2. See my *Human Identity and Bioethics* (Cambridge: Cambridge University Press, 2005) and Eric Olson, *The Human Animal* (New York: Oxford University Press, 1997).

3. See Jeff McMahan, *The Ethics of Killing* (New York: Oxford University Press, 2002), chaps. 2 and 3.

4. A central thesis of *Human Identity and Bioethics* is that appreciating this distinction is crucial in addressing a wide variety of issues in bioethics.

5. See David Benatar, *Better Never to Have Been?* (Oxford: Oxford University Press, 2006) and Seanna Shiffrin, "Wrongful Life, Procreative Responsibility, and the Significance of Harm," *Legal Theory* 5 (1999): 117–48.

6. The classic discussion of this problem is Derek Parfit, *Reasons and Persons* (Oxford: Clarendon, 1984), chap. 16.

2

Prenatal Moral Status and Ethics

Most human beings are created naturally through sexual reproduction. Some are created less naturally, with the assistance of reproductive technologies prior to implantation in a woman's uterus. And some are created in vitro for scientific purposes without any reproductive intent. Today, no ethical issue is more contentious than abortion, which involves the killing of an embryo or fetus. Not much less contentious are embryonic stem-cell research, research cloning, and other types of embryo research that involve the destruction of embryos. All of these issues provoke the question of how we should understand the moral status of prenatal human beings.

Let us use the term "prenatal human being" broadly to apply to any living but unborn member of our species. That would include the one-cell product of conception (fertilization)—the zygote—as well as what develops from the zygote, often referred to as the embryo in the early weeks after conception and later, when organs become apparent, as the fetus (although sometimes "fetus" is used to refer to the developing human organism throughout gestation). "Prenatal human beings" in our broad sense also includes living human organisms that are not expected to be born or even to enter a woman's uterus—in particular, embryos created artificially for research purposes.

How are we to understand the moral status of prenatal human beings? Do they matter morally in their own right, independently of their usefulness or their relations to people like you or me (postnatal human beings whose moral status and personhood are uncontested)? If they matter morally in their own right, how much do they matter? Do they have a right to life such that it is impermissible to kill them? If they lack such a right to life, does their status nevertheless ground a moral obligation not to destroy them for trivial purposes? To answer these questions, we need to know what underlies moral status. Why do those who are uncontroversially persons enjoy moral status—or, if the latter admits of degrees, full moral status? The answer will permit us to determine whether some or all prenatal human beings share this status. If they do, and if it is wrong to kill anyone with such status, this would appear to vindicate a "pro-life" or conservative approach to the ethics of abortion and embryo research. If they do not, that would presumably open the door to liberal approaches to these issues.

It is worth noting early on that the ethical issues of abortion and embryo research involve moral dimensions in addition to prenatal moral status. Abortion, for starters, involves the termination of unwanted pregnancies, which occur in women's bodies; and people have extensive rights to determine what happens to and within their bodies—at least as far as other people's actions and social policies (as opposed to natural forces like diseases) are concerned. Indeed, according to one school of thought we will consider, a woman's rights to bodily integrity and liberty are of such paramount importance that the fetus's moral status proves largely irrelevant to the ethics of abortion. This issue may also be understood to involve broader social issues such as gender roles, patriarchy, and freedom of conscience in a secular, pluralistic society. Meanwhile, the ethics of embryo research implicates issues of how taxpayers' money ought to be spent, embryo research being heavily dependent on public funding, as well as concerns about the possible commodification of prenatal human life and threats to traditional understandings of human procreation. The purpose here is not to provide an exhaustive catalogue of issues other than moral status that can and do come into play in discussions of abortion and ethical research. The purpose, rather, is to note some of them in order to avoid an oversimplified picture according to which prenatal moral status is all that matters in these discussions. At the same time, because it is widely believed that full moral status entails a right to life, and that the intentional destruction of an embryo or fetus would violate such a right (if it exists), it is no wonder that so many ethical discussions of these topics have centered on moral status. We will focus on prenatal moral status for much of the chapter before turning to other considerations that underlie some of the most powerful arguments in the ethical debates over abortion and embryo research.

The chapter's first major section will defend a tripartite framework for understanding prenatal moral status. This framework consists of (1) a view about our numerical identity, essence, and origins; (2) an account of the relevance of sentience to moral status; and (3) a version of the "time-relative interests account" of the harm of death. (All technical terms will be explained later.) As we will see, this framework supports relatively liberal views about abortion and embryo research. In the next section, I rebut what I take to be the three strongest arguments in favor of a pro-life approach. I also address what many consider the strongest argument for a liberal view of abortion—the Good Samaritan Argument—asking whether it clinches the case for a liberal position, and arguing that it does not. In the section that follows, I argue, perhaps surprisingly, that one might reasonably doubt the framework I have defended, that there are considerations that could lead a reasonable, well-informed person thinking entirely in secular terms to maintain a pro-life view. Thus, I argue for a sort of pluralism regarding prenatal moral status. In view of what I regard as a stalemate at the level of ontology (in particular, the issues of our essence and origins) and ethics, I redirect the discussion to the level of political philosophy and social policy. I argue that while a pro-life approach is reasonable, it rests on three assumptions: one about our essence and origins, another about the constancy of moral status throughout one's lifetime, and a third about the relationship between full moral status and the ethics of killing prenatal human beings. Because each of these assumptions is highly debatable, as demonstrated by the preceding discussion—and in view of women's interests in liberty and bodily integrity as well as biomedical researchers' interest in freedom of inquiry—I argue that ontological and ethical pluralism supports some sort of liberal approach to policy. In the final section, I sketch and defend such an approach to abortion and embryo research.

A FRAMEWORK FOR UNDERSTANDING PRENATAL MORAL STATUS

Those who are indisputably persons have full moral status. This status incorporates a right to life—by which I mean a nearly absolute moral protection against being intentionally or negligently killed that generally resists appeals to utility as justifications for killing. If zygotes, embryos, and fetuses share this moral status, that is presumably because (1) they are beings of our kind from the time of conception, and (2) a being of our kind has moral status for the entire duration of its existence. Let us first consider the issue underlying claim (1). When do beings like you and me come into existence?

Our Essence, Numerical Identity, and Origins

The question of when we come into being, or originate, is conceptually tied to the question of our essence: What are we human persons, most fundamentally? Which of our characteristics are so fundamental that their loss would entail that we literally go out of existence? Answering this question will tell us which properties have to be present for one of us to exist; one of us originates as soon as those essential properties appear. A related question is that of our numerical identity: Once we have come into being, what are the criteria for our continued existence, amid change, over time? What are our persistence conditions? (The concept of numerical identity is distinct from that of narrative identity, though scholars routinely confuse them in the bioethics and philosophical literature.[1] A person's narrative identity is something particular to her as an individual—namely, her self-concept or how she views herself as the subject of her implicit autobiography.[2])

Psychological Views and their Difficulties

One view of our essence, which we may call person essentialism, holds that we human persons are essentially persons and therefore could not exist at any time without being persons at that time.[3] Here persons are understood, roughly, as beings with the capacity for relatively complex forms of consciousness such as reasoning, intentional action, self-awareness, linguistic thought, and the like. (Hereafter, I will use the term "person" in this way. Because I do not assume that only persons have full moral status, this usage will not beg questions about the moral status of those classified as nonpersons.) According to person essentialism, you would not survive in an irreversible coma; the human organism that continues to breathe would not be you.

Elsewhere I have argued at length that this view is thoroughly implausible.[4] For one thing, it implies that you were never a newborn. Because newborns lack the capacity (as opposed to potential) for the sorts of consciousness associated with personhood, they are not persons, from which it follows—for the person essentialist—that no human person is numerically identical with any newborn of the past. I take it, however, that each of us was once a newborn. Another major problem with person essentialism is its difficulty accounting adequately for the relationship between any person and the human organism or animal associated with her. Here is one aspect of this problem: Since a person, on this view, has a time of origination and persistence conditions that differ from those of the associated human organism—the organism existing for the duration of biological life, the person existing only when the capacity for sufficiently complex forms of consciousness exists—the person, strictly speaking, is not an animal. This implies, contrary to scientifically informed common sense, that you are not an animal.[5]

More plausible than person essentialism is another psychological view of our essence, mind essentialism, which claims that we human persons are essentially minds: beings with the capacity for consciousness (that is, for at least some conscious states even if not those characteristic of persons).[6] Late fetuses and newborns are clearly sentient and therefore have states of consciousness, however primitive. So mind essentialism does not imply, implausibly, that we did not exist as newborns. It does imply, however, that we were never pre-sentient fetuses. While I find that dubious, many people do not, so this implication may not threaten the view. I suggest, though, that like person essentialism, mind essentialism lacks an adequate characterization of the person/human animal relationship; among its implications are again that, strictly speaking, you are not an animal. This in turn apparently implies that, as you read these words, there are two conscious beings sitting in your chair: you, the person or mind, and the associated animal, who (possessing a well-functioning brain) is certainly conscious. As far as conscious beings go, this seems one too many.

One who defends mind essentialism might claim that you are part of the animal associated with you—namely the brain (more precisely, the portions of the brain associated with consciousness).[7] But the brain seems capable of surviving death, whereas, on this view, you are not. Are you, then, a functioning brain, which goes out of existence at the irreversible loss of the capacity for consciousness? But it seems odd to identify the functioning brain—as distinct from the brain—as you. How could you be some organ only when it functions? Presumably you are a substance in the philosophical sense—something that bears properties—not a particular substance only when it has certain properties such as those of the brain that make consciousness possible. A proponent of mind essentialism might reply that the functioning brain is itself a substance, a substance distinct from the brain, but that claim, too, strains credibility. Might you instead be not the brain, but the mind understood as the conscious properties of the brain (or perhaps the physical properties of the brain that make consciousness possible)? That would imply that you are a set of properties, rather than a substance, a wildly counterintuitive thesis.

When the argumentative dust settles, I find mind essentialism less plausible than the view I defend, the biological view. But the biological view also faces challenges.[8] The balance of arguments is quite close, so mind essentialism, unlike person essentialism, should be considered a contender among views of our essence, numerical identity, and origins.

The Biological Approach

According to the biological view, we are essentially human organisms, or animals, so that we come into being whenever the relevant organism does, and we persist for the duration of biological life. When does the human organism that characteristically develops into a person originate? Many defenders of the pro-life view assume that the answer must be: at conception, the moment when sperm and egg unite, forming a new entity—the zygote—endowed with a full complement of human genes, the program that over time drives the emergence and growth of a human person.[9] I argue that this seemingly innocent assumption is highly questionable. True, at conception a new entity comes into being, and this being appears at first glance to persist through all the stages of gestation and post-natal life, but there are powerful reasons to doubt this appearance.[10]

For approximately two weeks after conception, the embryo can divide into two or more parts that go on to develop into separate human beings, and it can fuse with another embryo to constitute a new organism. Call this the case of division monozygotic twinning (ignoring the possibilities of triplets, quadruplets, etc.). The resulting embryos, from which identical twins derive, have virtually identical DNA. By contrast, "fraternal" twins, resulting from the fertilization of two eggs in one cycle, feature only the genetic similarity typical of ordinary siblings. Let us use the term "fusion" to refer to the unusual occurrence in which two embryos, fraternal twins, merge into one, a chimera. The chimera has two complete sets of DNA, which together determine (along with prenatal and postnatal environment) the individual's phenotype—observable characteristics such as eye color, height, and talents.

So, until about two weeks after conception, an embryo can divide into two and, in cases of fraternal twinning, two embryos can fuse into one. Arguably, then, the single-cell zygote is not really a human organism of the sort that we are—that is, one of us at an early stage. Perhaps it is more like living building material out of which one (or more) of us may emerge.

Consider any pair of adult identical twins and any adult chimera. The twins derived from the same zygote. If each human organism originated as a single-cell zygote, then each of twins came into being as the very same zygote. But this is an incoherent result. After all, the twins are numerically distinct from each other, so both cannot be identical to a single earlier zygote. (I make the standard assumption that identity is transitive: If A = B, and B = C, then A = C.) Meanwhile, no chimera could have originated from a single zygote because two such beings were needed to constitute her genome. Surely, she did not originate until fusion occurred; and the twins did not come into being until twinning took place. Neither chimeras nor identical twins could have originated at conception. (As we will see, one contending model of twinning somewhat complicates this claim.)

Now, it does not follow from these points that human beings who are neither identical twins nor chimeras did not originate at conception. Maybe different human beings originate at different stages of development. This is possible, but there is substantial reason to think that no human being comes into existence at conception.

In order to see why, it will be helpful to consider two models of how twinning occurs.[11] According to the division model, the more traditional understanding of twinning, a single embryo divides into two embryos roughly equal in size. According to the budding model, a blastomere (cell) leaves the original embryo and develops independently. We currently do not know which model is correct; perhaps each applies in some instances. If we originate at conception, what happens to the original human organism in twinning cases? If division occurs, then the original organism exists very briefly before vanishing at the time of twinning; whenever an embryo divides, a human organism of our kind goes out of existence. This coheres with the thesis that, while most human beings originate at conception, identical twins originate at the time of twinning. If budding occurs, on the other hand, the original human organism continues to exist despite losing a cell; that cell, which goes on to develop, would constitute a fresh human organism. So budding entails that one twin originates at conception whereas the other comes into being a bit later. These are implications of the thesis that we—that is, most of us—originate at conception.

Some will find it odd that at least some twins and the rest of us, who are of the same basic kind, should originate at different stages of prenatal development. More important than the possible sense of oddity is a related, deeper concern: that the early embryo is, arguably, less like a single, unified organism than like a colony of organisms loosely conjoined by the zona pellucida (the membrane that keeps the cells together). To develop this idea, we need to bear in mind what an organism is. Organisms are characterized by internal complexity featuring interdependent subsystems and the drawing of energy from the environment to maintain internal organization and resist entropy; and no organism (unlike, say, an organ) is part of a larger biological entity. Organisms can consist of a single cell because even a cell features great internal complexity and interdependent subsystems. Amoebas are such organisms. So is the single-cell zygote. Furthermore, the zygote is human as opposed to, say, feline or canine. The question is whether it is a human organism of the same kind that you and I instantiate.

For the first few cell divisions, according to the present school of thought, the embryo functions less like a single integrated, energy-using unit of the sort we call an organism than like a collection of single-cell organisms contingently stuck together. That is precisely why twinning and fusion remain possible. After the sperm penetrates the egg, their respective sets of chromosomes remain separate for about a day. Contrary to popular belief, fertilization is completed at the two-cell stage.[12] Two further divisions in the next couple of days result in an eight-cell embryo. Significantly, each of the eight cells retains the potential, if separated, to produce a human organism like you or me. Thus far there is no specialization of cells to perform distinct tasks; nor is there significant interaction or integration among them. In that sense, they are not functioning as a single, integrated organism. Rather, they are tantamount to a colony of eight contingently joined zygotes.

Cell differentiation begins, the argument continues, at the 16-cell stage, as the outer cells begin to transform into what will become the placenta. Division continues as the embryo travels through the fallopian tube, entering the uterus about five days after (the beginning of) fertilization. Two or three days later, it penetrates the uterine wall, establishing connections with the mother's blood supply. But the middle cells have not differentiated and the embryo could still divide spontaneously into two viable organisms. On day 14 or 15, some middle cells differentiate, and it is now determined which cells will form part of the placenta and which will become part of the fetus. Within a day, in the fetal portion, a column of cells differentiates into the "primitive streak," the precursor to the spinal cord. Spontaneous twinning is now impossible. There undeniably exists a human organism that functions as a single integrated unit. From the standpoint of the biological view of our essence and identity, this organism is a being of our kind. In other words, it is a being that can grow into—become— what is indisputably a human person.

So, once spontaneous twinning is precluded and every portion of the embryo is differentiated at about two weeks after conception, one of us exists. But maybe we should judge that we emerge earlier, when differentiation begins at the 16-cell stage. Rather than drawing a line marking our time of origination, I tentatively advance two theses: (1) None of us existed, prior to the 16-cell stage, as a completely undifferentiated embryo (a portion of which later differentiates into the placenta); and (2) By the time twinning is precluded and all embryonic parts are differentiated, one of us has originated. Possibly we come into existence somewhat gradually over several days rather than at a single moment.

Having presented this understanding of our origins, from the backdrop of a biological view of our essence and identity, I must acknowledge the respectability of another biologically based understanding of our origins. This alternative receives motivation from the thesis that there is significant integration very soon, perhaps even immediately, after conception. Suggesting this possibility is a report of several experiments involving mouse embryos, the upshot of which is the appearance in mice of cell differentiation as early as the two-cell stage.[13] Might human embryos also feature such early, or even earlier, integration and differentiation? Some have argued affirmatively, citing recent scientific sources. One team of authors, for example, has contended that "there must be some kind of exchange of information both within the single-cell zygote and within the multiple-cell zygote. . . ."[14] This possibility should not be ignored.

At the same time, even if there proves to be some integration of functioning among various parts of the zygote, it seems fair to ask, "How much integration and differentiation are sufficient for the zygote to be appropriately classified as an organism that can grow into one of us (entailing numerical identity between the zygote and later person) as opposed to an organism that merely precedes and furnishes the building blocks for one of us?" After all, there are insufficient integration and differentiation of the zygote/early embryo to preclude spontaneous twinning and fusion. And much of this organism will go on to form the placenta rather than the later embryo. So the facts of embryology alone may not settle the issue of when we originate. Some degree of interpretation may be necessary.

We conclude this discussion of our essence, identity, and origins with the first prong of a tripartite framework for understanding prenatal moral status—and some uncertainty about one end of this prong. I have recommended, and briefly defended, a biological view according to which we are essentially human organisms or animals such that our persistence conditions are biological: the continuation of a single life. For those who accept the biological view, there is uncertainty about our origins. We come into being as pre-sentient embryos, but when exactly? The view I suggest places our origins somewhere between the 16-cell stage and around two weeks post-gestation when twinning is precluded and differentiation is fully established. Another respectable view is that we originate much closer to, and perhaps at, the time of conception.

Sentience, Interests, and Moral Status

On the biological view, we originate within the first two weeks or so of gestation. Do we have full moral status as soon as we originate? We do if we have this status throughout the entirety of our existence. But we cannot simply assume that this is the case, so we need to consider the basis of our moral status. What is it about us, or about any beings with moral status, that confers it? We will begin by considering moral status in general before introducing the possibility of degrees of moral status.

THE APPEAL TO SPECIES
In light of moral tradition and current practices, it may seem natural to judge that the basis of moral status is being human in the sense of species membership. On this view, all and only members of Homo sapiens have moral status—and they have it precisely because they are members of this species. However natural it may seem to think along these lines, this position proves remarkably implausible. For one thing, it is hardly credible that a biological category such as species could furnish the criterion of moral status. If species itself—as opposed to characteristics normally associated with a species—is the basis of moral status, then a person who was not Homo sapiens (say, a member of a now-extinct hominid species, an extraordinary animal, or a space alien) would not qualify. This is hardly plausible. Why should our species be so special?

Moreover, if membership in a biological grouping is supposed to make all the difference, why species rather than a more general category such as genus, family, or order? Why only Homo sapiens and not any other hominid species, or other primates, and so forth? Or why not a biological grouping more specific than species? For example, one might claim that only male members of our species have moral status. It would be useless to reply that women and girls are just as intelligent, self-aware, and sensitive as men and boys, because the working assumption is that it is a biological grouping, not some associated characteristic, that underlies moral status. And, unlike distinctions of race, distinctions of sex—male and female—have about as much claim to being biologically real as species distinctions do.[15] There is no good reason to believe that membership in our species is the basis of moral status.[16]

THE PERSONHOOD VIEW

A more plausible thesis is that some characteristic or a set of characteristics associated with our species provides the basis of moral status. The paradigm bearers of moral status, after all, are persons, where persons are understood as beings with the capacity for sufficiently complex forms of consciousness; normal post-infancy human beings are generally assumed to make the grade. Persons, moreover, can be accountable to each other, each person having obligations to other persons. If all and only persons have moral status, then there is a neat congruence between (1) beings who have moral status and (2) beings who bear moral responsibility—moral agents or persons. For these reasons, it is understandable that many people might believe personhood to be the basis for moral status.

Nevertheless, like the species-based view, the personhood view proves deeply problematic. For one thing, it has difficulties with the moral status of human nonpersons. Consider so-called nonparadigm humans—human beings who, due to genetic anomaly or environmental insult, do not have (even potentially) the mental capacities that constitute personhood. No matter how personhood is defined, so long as it is defined in terms of mental capacities that are supposed to distinguish us from cats and dogs, some humans—including the most severely retarded and the most severely demented—will not qualify as persons. Yet it is incredible to think that they, at least those who remain sentient (capable of having feelings), lack moral status; surely they are not fair game for dangerous, nontherapeutic experiments, forced labor, or consumption by cannibals. There must be something wrong, therefore, with any view whose criteria for moral status imply that these individuals fall on the wrong side of the line. Moreover, it is not so clear that the personhood view adequately handles the moral status of ordinary infants. Newborns are not yet persons in the relevant sense, but it seems pretty obvious that they have moral status. To be sure, they are potential persons—meaning that in due course they will develop into persons—but so are embryos (at least after twinning is precluded) and fetuses. Only those who hold that these prenatal human beings have the moral status of persons can assert, on the basis of potential, that infants do as well.[17] I suggest that the personhood view's difficulties with nonparadigm humans, and perhaps ordinary infants, reflects an untenable criterion for moral status.

A second major problem for the personhood view is that it seems unable to account adequately for the wrongness of cruelty to animals. Horses are not persons, yet it is wrong to abuse them. Can the wrongness of cruelty to horses (or other sentient animals) be fully explained in terms of human interests? Many horses are legally owned by particular persons, so harming the horse damages someone's property—which is generally wrong. And many people are upset by cruelty to horses, so to abuse these creatures is to offend these people's sensibilities. But these points about human interests do not get to the heart of the matter. To abuse a horse is to harm her, greatly, for no good reason—and, intuitively, that fact by itself seems sufficient to explain the wrong. Accordingly, to abuse an animal who was no one's property, and about whom few if any people cared, would seem wrong, a point that is not accounted for if only persons have moral status. There is compelling reason to believe that at least some nonpersons—some human, some nonhuman—have moral status.

Do all Living Things have Moral Status?
One might conjecture that all living things have moral status. This thesis would avoid the implausible narrowness of the personhood criterion, but at the expense of excessive breadth. In addition to covering persons and clearly sentient animals, it would cover the most primitive animals, whose nervous systems seem incapable of sustaining (conscious) sensations, as well as plants, fungi, and bacteria. Why should anyone believe these insentient creatures have moral status? Given their lack of sentience, in what sense can they be harmed? It is a plausible thesis that only sentient creatures—beings who can experience feelings—can be harmed or benefited and therefore have interests.[18]

Some argue, however, that all living creatures have interests grounded in biological needs—for whatever is necessary to survive, maintain health, and perhaps reproduce—and that to thwart these interests by damaging or killing the life in question is to harm it.[19] The notion of biological needs helps us to understand how something might have interests despite never experiencing feelings such as pain and pleasure. We may say that a flower needs water, sunlight, and soil conducive to growth even though the flower has no mind and therefore does not care about these things. After all, if the biological needs are not met, the flower will wilt and die. "Conditions necessary to sustain life and health" is a tolerably clear standard for determining the interests of a living being.

But is this standard plausible? Why should we judge that a lifeform has an interest in remaining alive if that being does not care about its life? It certainly does not take an interest in its life, or anything for which the life is a precondition, because, being permanently insentient, it cannot take an interest in anything. For this reason, it seems that the mindless lifeform has no stake in its own life or anything else.

One might reply that a flower's life in some sense matters to the flower, because, if it languishes or dies, it loses its physical integrity. But why should that matter—in any sense that can be unpacked in terms of the flower's interests as opposed to the interests, say, of people who like flowers? If we assert that a flower needs to stay alive to retain its physical integrity, we should also judge that a lawn mower needs to be oiled to maintain its integrity and not break down, and a house needs to be well maintained for the same reason. Yet lawn mowers and houses do not have interests.

One might reply that living things are natural entities whereas lawnmowers and houses are artificial, and that only natural entities can have interests. But this reply is not persuasive. Surely an advanced artificial-intelligence system that (or who) achieved consciousness and feelings would have interests despite being artificial. Moreover, many natural but nonliving systems such as waterfalls, planets, and galaxies have structures that could be considered the bases of their integrity, yet no one would claim that they therefore have interests. Physical integrity or the "need" to maintain structure is not sufficient to ground interests.

Is there another possible basis for saying that plants and insentient animals, as living things, have interests and therefore moral status? One might claim that all and only living things have a naturally given end—to grow and live in a characteristic way—and that this end gives rise to interests. But one might as well say, absurdly, that rivers have a naturally given end to keep flowing, that black holes have a naturally given end to absorb and compress everything within their reach into singularities, and that rivers and black holes therefore have interests in whatever conditions are necessary for them to fulfill their respective ends. These reflections suggest that there is no credible basis for claiming that interests and therefore moral status are grounded in biological needs, independently of conscious experience.

Consider, then, a different possible basis for the claim that all living things have moral status: the view that all life commands our respect, irrespective of whether it has interests and can be benefitted or harmed. Personally, I tend to agree that we should have an attitude of awe or reverence for living things, but I think that this attitude should extend to all of nature. As we just saw, living things are not distinguished from the rest of nature by possession of interests, because many living creatures lack interests. It seems, then, that whatever respect is appropriately directed to living things as such, or to living things as part of nature, must be due to some value-based factor (perhaps aesthetic) other than moral status.

The Sentience View

Our reflections on moral status suggest that (1) not only persons and human beings have moral status, and (2) not all living things have it. Some nonhuman nonpersons have moral status because they can be affected by the actions of moral agents in ways that they, the nonpersons, experience and presumably care about insofar as their quality of life is affected. In that way, they can be benefited or harmed. The reason why not all living things have moral status is that many of them have no subjective experience and therefore no quality of life and no interests. These observations strongly suggest a basis for moral status that has been embraced by many theorists and that I have defended at length in another place: the sentience view.[20] According to this view, sentient beings—who by definition are capable of having feelings—are precisely those beings who have interests and can be harmed or benefited (in any sense that might be morally important); all and only such beings are of direct moral concern. That I help a person affects her interests and, for this reason, matters morally. That I abuse a horse thwarts her interest in avoiding suffering and, for this reason, matters morally. That I kill bacteria with an antibiotic or smash a rock does not affect the interests of the bacteria or rock, which lack interests, and does not matter morally—unless my action importantly affects the interests of persons or other sentient beings.

So the sentience view has several advantages. It has no difficulty explaining why not only human persons, but also (sentient) human nonpersons have moral status and should not be abused or exploited. It straightforwardly explains the wrongness of cruelty to animals who are capable of suffering from cruelty. (One cannot really be cruel to an amoeba or plant.) More generally, it squares very well with our intuitions about morally important harms and benefits. And, if there is something right about the personhood view of moral status, the sentience view can partly accommodate it: One can hold both that all sentient beings have moral status and that persons have special moral status.

In virtue of its conceptual tie to interests, the sentience view connects plausibly with two leading types of ethical theory. First, it connects well with consequentialism, the general approach according to which the rightness or wrongness of our actions is a function of their consequences. Such theories need an account of individual well-being to cash out how the consequences of actions affect us in ways that matter. The concept of an interest—as a component of well-being—serves this role well. Second, the sentience approach fits well with rights theories, according to which individuals have certain rights, understood as moral protections or claims that are not (or only rarely) to be violated even in pursuit of good ends. To what do individuals have rights? This a matter of great dispute, of course, but one safe claim is that A can have a right to X only if A has an interest in X. We might add that it is our most vital, central, or important interests that provide the basis for rights. In any case, interests provide the content or conceptual material for a well-developed account of rights just as they provide the content for a well-developed account of individual well-being.[21]

Thus, the second prong of the recommended three-part framework for understanding prenatal moral status is this thesis: Beings with moral status are precisely those beings who have interests, which are closely connected with sentience. But what is the precise connection between sentience and interests? Some who adopt the sentience view hold that sentience is necessary and sufficient for having interests and therefore for having moral status,[22] but I'm not so sure. Based on our reflections, we may confidently assert that sentience is sufficient for interests and moral status (a claim that implies that late fetuses have moral status). But is sentience necessary? One might assume so, considering such cases as paintings, planets, plants, and protozoa. But what if a non-sentient being has the potential to grow into a sentient being? Might it have an interest in realizing this potential, despite being presently unable to appreciate it? We must consider this possibility.

Potential Sentience and Time-Relative Interests

Persons have moral status and so do other sentient beings. What about beings that are potentially sentient beings or persons? Obviously, it does not follow from the fact that A is potentially X, which has a certain status, that A already has that status. For example, it does not follow from the fact that I am potentially Professor Emeritus that I already have this status, on the basis of which I can claim certain privileges such as commandeering an office without doing any work. In discussions of moral status, liberal scholars often make much of this logical point, but doing so provides little help in understanding the real issue concerning potential.

The real issue concerns not potential in general, but the prenatal human being's potential—for sentience, personhood, or both. Taking our cue from the sentience view, and accepting that a fetus ordinarily becomes sentient late in pregnancy (probably no earlier than the beginning of the third trimester[23]), we can reformulate our question as follows: Does the pre-sentient human being already have interests on the basis of what it can become? Can it have interests before it has a nervous system capable of producing states of consciousness?

Many thinkers, especially liberals, are likely to answer in the negative and to endorse:

The View that Sentience is Necessary. Pre-sentient fetuses cannot have interests. To have an interest is to have a stake in something; it is to be susceptible of being made better off or worse off. But to have a stake or to be so susceptible requires that one care about certain things, have preferences, or at least have sensations that are experienced as pleasant or unpleasant—in other words, a quality of life. True, we sometimes have interests in things that we don't care about, prefer, or even know about—for example, an interest in learning that one has an inheritance from a distant relative. But in such cases, our interest is ultimately a function of things we do care about, prefer, etc. such as having enough money and obtaining what is legally ours. Having no conscious life at all, a pre-sentient fetus has no carings or concerns that can be the basis of such interests.

This is a powerful argument. I think it may be correct. But I am not at all sure, because there is another way of looking at the matter that strikes me as equally cogent:

The View that Potential is Sufficient. Imagine that a baby has just been born to loving parents who are well-positioned to care for her. The baby has one striking anomaly but is otherwise perfectly healthy: Due to a problem with a portion of her brainstem, she has never been conscious. She can gain consciousness only if a simple medical procedure is performed. With this procedure, the baby can acquire a mental life that will very likely develop normally. Undoubtedly, it is in this baby's interest to have the procedure performed so that she can become conscious. Some believe that any conscious life—or sentience[24]—is intrinsically valuable (assuming the subject isn't terribly miserable). Others believe that, while sentience automatically gives rise to interests, it is only the conscious life of a person that is intrinsically valuable (assuming, again, the quality of life isn't too low). Either way, this baby has the relevant potential. It would be a terrible loss for her not to have the procedure and thereby lose the riches of the life she can have. In the same way, a fetus with the same potential has an interest in remaining alive. Whatever it is about human lives (of tolerable quality) that makes them so valuable for their subjects, a fetus stands to gain such a treasure if she is able to live. It is irrelevant that the fetus, like the baby, cannot now appreciate this possible future of value. It is relevant that the fetus is a creature whose endowment naturally inclines it to develop in such a way that it will eventually achieve sentience and later the mental life of a person.

This, too, is a powerful argument—about as powerful, I think, as the View that Sentience is Necessary.

Political liberals tend to overlook or underestimate arguments along the lines of the View that Potential is Sufficient. One reason, surely, is a desire not to threaten a woman's presumed right to abortion. Another reason, I think, is a tendency to trivialize the notion of potential. Critics of pro-life arguments often claim that appeals to potential are illegitimate because they would absurdly legitimate claims of moral status on behalf of sperm, ova, and somatic cells (which, in principle, can be cloned).[25] But the relevant potential is not mere logical possibility or even factual possibility. Rather, it is natural potentiality, which is possessed by members of a kind of thing whose natural development involves realizing the relevant potential. Another error is to think that for A to be potentially a B, it is enough that A can become a piece of a B. I have heard it said that a piece of dust has the potential to become a statue because the former could end up being combined with other particles in the construction of a statue. Not much more plausible is the claim that a sperm cell could become one of us. No, a sperm cell can combine with an ovum to constitute a new entity with a full complement of human genes; depending on the correct view of our origins as discussed earlier, either this entity can become one of us or it can provide the material from which one of us emerges when there is sufficient integration and differentiation. To do justice to pro-life thinking, we need to appreciate that its proponents have a special sense of "potential" in mind when they appeal to a fetus' potential. I do not mean that such appeals should be accepted uncritically, just that they should be understood on the terms of those who advance them rather than misconstrued into straw targets that are easily knocked over. Properly understood, the appeal to a fetus' potential is part of a powerful argument, as displayed in the View that Potential is Sufficient.

Does a pre-sentient fetus have an interest in staying alive, an interest based on its potential to enjoy a valuable sort of existence? I just do not know. If the answer were clearly No, then prenatal status would be greatly clarified: Fetuses would lack moral status until they achieved sentience. This result would greatly simplify the ethics of abortion and embryo research. But suppose, now, that the answer is Yes: The pre-sentient fetus has an interest in remaining alive. For the sake of argument, I will assume that this view is correct. I will argue that, even on this pro-life-friendly assumption, there are powerful grounds for denying that this fetal interest supports a fetal right to life.

These grounds stem from the time-relative interest account (TRIA) of the harm of death.[26] This account is motivated by observations about what we believe about the harm of death in different cases. How much is one harmed by death? It might seem logical to assume that the magnitude of the harm of death should be determined solely in terms of how much good life one loses (where "how much good life" takes into account both quality and quantity of life). From this whole-lifetime perspective, the younger one is, other things—quality of life, expected lifespan—being equal, the more prudential value or good one loses from death. This implies that a pre-sentient fetus is harmed a bit more by death than is an infant, who is harmed more by death than a 10- or 25-year-old. But precisely the opposite seems correct: Other things equal, death seems to harm a 10- or 25-year-old more than it harms an infant, and an infant at least a bit more than a pre-sentient fetus. We may well regard the death of the pre-sentient fetus as unfortunate for it; people's intuitions seem to vary on this point (as reflected in the clash between the View that Sentience is Necessary and the View that Potential is Sufficient). Most of us would probably consider the infant's death a major misfortune for him. By contrast, we regard the death of a 10- or 25-year-old as utterly tragic for the victim—and in a way that fetal and infantile death cannot be for its victim. Note: The claim is not that others are likely to mourn an infant's death less than that of a 10- or 25-year-old, a claim that can be explained by the family's having invested more, emotionally and otherwise, in the older victim. The present claim concerns the harm of death to the one who dies.

So the view that the harm of death is simply a function of total lost pruden-tial good generates implausible implications about the comparative harm of death in different cases.[27] Our reflections suggest that the harm of death is a function not only of lost opportunities for valuable life, but of another factor as well. Simply stated, the second factor according to the TRIA is the extent to which one is psychologically connected with one's possible future life.

The TRIA discounts the harm of death to its victim, at the time of death, for any weakness in the psychological unity that would have connected the victim at that time with herself in the future. In this way, it denies that numerical identity—being one and the same individual over time—is the only relation that an indi-vidual has to herself over time that matters prudentially; psychological unity over time also matters. The degree of psychological unity in a life, or over a stretch of time, is a function of (1) the amount of internal reference between earlier and later mental states (e.g., memories of past experiences, anticipations of future experiences), (2) the proportion of the subject's mental life that is sustained over the stretch of time in question, and (3) the richness of the mental life.[28] When the psychological unity that would have bound an individual at the time of death to herself in the future, had she lived, is weak, death matters less prudentially—for that individual—at that time.

The TRIA steers a plausible middle course between two polar positions, as we can see by considering the death of an infant. On a desire-satisfaction ac-count of the harm of death, one is harmed by death only if one desires to remain alive, or not to die, but such a desire seems impossible within the primitive conceptual repertoire of infants. So the desire-satisfaction account implies, implausibly, that normal human infants are not harmed by death. Contrast the view that construes the harm of death in terms of lost opportunities for valuable future experiences, while assuming a whole-lifetime perspective. This view implies that death typically harms an infant more than a child, adolescent, or young adult. This, at least to my mind, seems highly implausible. Steering between the implications of these two views, the TRIA suggests that death significantly harms the infant but not nearly as much as it harms the child, adolescent, or young adult. In addition to delivering this plausible verdict, the TRIA explains precisely what factor justifies discounting the disvalue of death, in cases like the infant's, as it would be understood from a whole-lifetime perspective: degree of psychological unity over time. The desire-satisfaction view is correct that caring about or appreciating (and therefore desiring) one's future is relevant to the harm of death, but wrong that one who does not appreciate or desire one's future life loses nothing from having that future snatched away. The whole-lifetime approach is right that appreciating one's future is not necessary for having a stake in that future, but incorrect in thinking that such appreciation is irrelevant to the harm of death. The TRIA, meanwhile, gets right what the polar views get right while avoiding their errors.

So the third prong of my tripartite framework for understanding prenatal moral status is the TRIA. How does it help us? Recall that we encountered a stalemate between the View that Sentience is Necessary and the View that Potential is Sufficient. For the sake of argument, we assumed that the latter was correct: The pre-sentient fetus has an interest in remaining alive. The significance of the TRIA is to show that any such interest must be very weak in comparison with a person's interest in remaining alive. Persons, in anything like ordinary circumstances, have a profound stake in staying alive, continued life being a foundation for the experiences, relationships, accomplishments, and so on that make one's life valuable for one. Persons also, more or less by definition, have deep psychological unity over time. Infants have much less, sentient fetuses precious little. To put it starkly, pre-sentient fetuses have no psychological unity with future stages of their lives because, prior to sentience, they have no psychology. Thus, even if we grant that the pre-sentient fetus has an interest—a prudential stake—in remaining alive, the TRIA implies that this interest is very weak. What the pre-sentient fetus stands to lose is enormous, but its lack of psychological life and therefore the lack of psychological unity between itself now and possible future stages of itself entail a weak time-relative interest in remaining alive. (A less generous interpretation, from the standpoint of the TRIA, would be that the pre-sentient fetus' lack of psychological life implies that this creature cannot have any time-relative interest in its future; in mathematical terms, where one of the factors is 0, the product must be 0.) So death is not a great harm for the pre-sentient fetus, suggesting little basis for attributing a right to life to it. This assumes, naturally, that a right to life depends on a strong interest in remaining alive, but that assumption seems entirely reasonable. Rights are grounded in strong interests.

This completes my defense of a tripartite framework for understanding prenatal moral status: (1) a biological view of our numerical identity, essence, and origins; (2) a view about the connections between interests, sentience, and moral status; and (3) the TRIA, which bears importantly on the moral status of pre-sentient fetuses. If this framework is substantially correct, it has implications for the ethics of abortion and embryo research that are at least moderately liberal, for it would imply that embryos and presentient fetuses have very little (if any) moral status in comparison with persons. But it is one thing to defend a framework, especially when, as here, the defense is relatively brief; it is another thing to make a compelling case for the framework. In an effort to make my case more compelling, I will turn to what I believe to be the strongest arguments in favor of a pro-life position and attempt to show that they are unpersuasive.

REPLYING TO THE STRONGEST PRO-LIFE ARGUMENTS

The Future-Like-Ours Argument

The Future-Like-Ours Argument (FLOA) has become the most celebrated anti-abortion argument in the English-speaking philosophical literature. Its celebrity is due, I think, partly to its quality, but also to the fact that its chief proponent, Don Marquis, is a politically liberal atheist who presumably lacks a conservative or religious agenda.[29] As we will see, the FLOA has much in common with the View that Potential is Sufficient.

The FLOA proceeds as follows. Why is it wrong, in ordinary circumstances, to kill paradigm persons like you or me? The fundamental reason is that killing us would deprive of us valuable futures, which would include all our personal projects, enjoyments, meaningful activities, and other valued experiences that are plausibly believed to make human life valuable in ordinary circumstances. This account of the wrongness of killing persons explains why we regard killing as such a terrible crime; it also accommodates our belief that death ordinarily harms the individual who dies. Meanwhile, it avoids certain difficulties of other leading accounts of the wrongness of killing persons, such as the desire-satisfaction account. Further, this approach plausibly implies that, since killing infants would (ordinarily) deprive them of valuable futures—futures like ours—infanticide is (at least normally) wrong. By contrast, accounts that base the wrongness of killing persons on their special moral status as persons—beings with the capacity for relatively complex forms of consciousness—struggle to explain the commonsense judgment that infanticide is normally wrong.

Now, the FLOA continues, consider fetuses (using the term broadly to refer to prenatal human organisms at any stage of development). A human fetus is an individual that can normally, if permitted to live, develop into a person who has the sorts of experiences we value so highly. So the fetus has a future like ours, making abortion comparable to the killing of paradigm persons: wrong in at least ordinary circumstances. This is a substantial moral argument against abortion that is free of religious assumptions, equivocation on the moral and descriptive senses of such terms as "human being" and "person," and question-begging appeals to potential.

When exactly does the FLOA first apply? In asserting that the fetus has a future like ours, the argument assumes that the fetus can develop into a paradigm person and, conversely, that each of us was once a fetus. So the FLOA applies whenever a human organism of our kind comes into existence. Our earlier discussion of our origins tentatively suggested that we come into existence at least a few days and no later than about two weeks after conception; it also acknowledged the respectability of the view that we come into existence as early as conception. If the FLOA is sound (whenever it first applies), it has far-reaching implications for prenatal moral status—and, if the latter is the primary consideration in the ethics of abortion, then for that issue as well. (Depending on when it first applies and what sort of embryo research is in question, it may or may not have far-reaching implications for the ethics of embryo research.)

Acceptance of the TRIA of the harm of death suggests that the FLOA is unsound. For the latter assumes that numerical identity is the sole basis for prudential concern for what most matters in our continued existence, suggesting that evaluation of a fetus' future should be made from a whole-lifetime perspective. From this perspective, of course, abortion (ordinarily) entails an enormous loss, the loss of a future like ours. On this basis, the FLOA infers that the fundamental consideration underlying the wrongness of killing paradigm persons also applies in the case of abortion. But in the previous section it was argued that the TRIA was a better account of the harm of death than the view presupposed by the FLOA. Fetuses, especially pre-sentient fetuses—the vast majority of fetuses aborted—have only weak (if any) time-relative interests in remaining alive. Thus, even if fetuses have a future like ours, the FLOA does not show that killing them is comparable to killing a paradigm person, or that fetuses have a right to life.

The Appeal to the Practical Necessity of Early Moral Protection

A second argument, which I call the Appeal to the Practical Necessity of Early Moral Protection, contends that we have full moral status for the full duration of our existence.[30] Coupled with the biological view of our essence and identity, it entails that the prenatal human being has full moral status from the moment of its origination (which, for the sake of simplicity, we will here assume to be conception). With the help of a third assumption—that a fetus' having full moral status would entail that it may not be intentionally killed—the Appeal to the Practical Necessity of Early Moral Protection supplies a substantial moral argument against abortion and (on the conception view of our origins) against embryo research.

The argument begins by noting that each of us who is able to consider this issue rightly holds herself to have full moral status. It then argues that it would be irrational for any of us—any person—to deny that she had full moral status at some earlier point in her existence. Why would this be irrational? As Alfonso Gomez-Lobo explains the idea, "Inviolability [full moral status] now without inviolability at previous stages entails that I would risk not being alive now. It would have been morally permissible to destroy me in the past so that my later inviolability would be worthless."[31] The idea is that the claim of present inviolability and the denial of earlier inviolability are somehow contradictory, and that, to avoid contradiction, we must maintain that every person is inviolable for the duration of her existence. But what kind of contradiction is supposedly involved? There is no logical contradiction, because the conjunction of "I now have full moral status" and "At some earlier time during my existence I did not have full moral status" cannot be resolved into the form of P and not P, as any logical contradiction can. Rather, the alleged contradiction, or absurdity, is practical: It would be absurd from the standpoint of practical reasoning to advance this conjunction of claims. Why? It is absurd, allegedly, to say that it would in the past have been permissible to destroy a being who later, if permitted to live, would have a moral status that makes such destruction impermissible. Yet, when I focus on this supposedly absurd statement, I perceive no absurdity. It may help in this context to highlight the distinction between what is permissible from an ethical standpoint and what is desirable from a prudential standpoint.

Consider an analogy. Marcie is glad to be alive, despite a rocky childhood. Her childhood was rocky because her parents lacked any good sense about how to raise children. In fact, Marcie can honestly say that her parents were far too immature to marry responsibly. They should not have married and certainly should not have had children. Yet, if they had not done these things, Marcie would not exist. So she judges that her parents did something wrong in marrying and having children, yet she is glad, self-interestedly, that they did so because she is glad she's alive. Is that contradictory or absurd? Not at all. From an impartial, ethical standpoint, Marcie judges that her parents failed to meet appropriate criteria for when people ought to feel free to marry and have children. From a partial, self-regarding standpoint, she values their actions as means to her current existence, which she values. While her position is likely to be psychologically awkward, it is certainly coherent and free from absurdity.

Returning to the central issue, can I consider myself presently inviolable and deny that I was inviolable in the earliest stages of existence? Yes, I can. My present full moral status entails that it would be wrong—extraordinary circumstances aside—for another to kill me. If I lacked this status as a fetus, then it would have been permissible for my mother to have an abortion, which would have killed me. I am glad that she did not because, like Marcie and most other people, I am glad to be alive. But I do not deny that it might have been permissible for me to have been aborted—say, if my mother had realistically judged that going to term and having another child would pose an overwhelming burden on her or the family. Partially and self-interestedly, I am glad that I was permitted to develop into a being with full moral status. But gladness does not entail entitlement. Impartially, I grant the possibility that this being could have been permissibly destroyed prior to acquiring full moral status. Moreover, present entitlement not to be killed does not entail past entitlement to enjoy conditions necessary for me to enjoy my present entitlement. Stated differently, present entitlement not to be killed does not entail present entitlement not to have been killed. So there is no contradiction or absurdity. Perhaps any feeling of a practical contradiction here trades on a conflation of ethical and prudential standpoints, which are distinct perspectives whose appropriate criteria of evaluation sometimes diverge.

The Appeal to Our Essence and Kind Membership

The third of what I take to be the three most powerful pro-life argument appeals to our membership in a kind defined by our essence, and the natural potentiality of members of this kind. The argument can be reconstructed as follows:

1. You and I have full moral status.
2. We have this status because of our essence, which determines our kind.
3. We are essentially human organisms—a kind endowed (essentially) with a rational nature.
4. Human organisms come into existence at conception.
Therefore,
5. We have full moral status from the time of conception.[32]

Like the Appeal to the Practical Necessity of Early Moral Protection, the present argument begins with the uncontroversial assumption that you and I, and paradigm persons generally, have full moral status. It further assumes a version of the biological view of our essence and identity, but adds the claim that human organisms are essentially rational. As for our origins, it assumes that we come into existence at conception—an assumption I will grant here, again, for simplicity's sake. The main vulnerabilities in this argument are two assumptions: the second part of 3 (call it 3b), the claim that our kind is essentially, therefore necessarily, rational; and premise 2, that our moral status is grounded in our essence and kind membership.

These two assumptions are importantly connected. Suppose the argument dropped 3b, asserting that we are essentially human organisms without claiming that we are essentially rational. One who, like me, accepted this assertion could hold that we are only characteristically rational, allowing that some human beings are not rational. Moreover, one could claim that this characteristic rationality is a trait that develops, gradually, after birth. It is certainly not true, one might argue, that we are rational at the time of conception—when we do not even have brains.

The Appeal to Our Essence and Kind Membership needs the assumption that all human organisms are rational by nature, and therefore rational regardless of how cognitively abnormal or damaged, and rational from the moment of conception. Without this assumption, given the traditional understanding (which pro-life thinkers accept) that personhood is necessary for full moral status, there would be no basis for saying that all members of our species—including the unborn and the severely cognitively disabled—enjoy this status. Persons are rational animals, the thinking goes, revealing its Aristotelean flavor. They are part of nature but their endowment, which includes rationality, distinguishes them from the rest of nature.

While it will strike many people as obvious that fetuses are not rational, since they evidently lack any capacity to reason, proponents of the present argument claim that fetuses actually have the capacity, in the form of natural potentiality, to reason. This capacity is part of their nature and simply needs to unfold with time. As Patrick Lee puts it, " . . . there is a sense in which human embryos and fetuses also have the capacity for higher mental functions. . . . They are members of a natural kind—a biological species—whose members, if not prevented by some extrinsic cause, in due course develop the immediately exercisable capacity for such mental functions."[33] So potentiality is involved. It is the potentiality to develop a certain kind of mental life that prominently includes rationality.[34]

Many will remain skeptical that fetuses, infants, or those human beings whose cognitive impairments prevent them from manifesting the mental life characteristic of persons are nevertheless rational. Doubts may be most acute in the case of the latter group because they cannot develop in such a way as to be able to reason, even if they are of a natural kind whose members characteristically develop this ability. But let us set aside the dubious claim that human organisms are essentially rational.[35] Let us focus instead on premise 2, that our moral status is determined by our essence and kind.

Our moral status must be based on something. Premise 2 states that the basis is membership in a kind determined by our essence. But other possible bases have been suggested as well. For example, it was argued earlier that the basis for moral status is the possession of interests. Now, a pro-life position can accept that having interests is necessary for moral status, because it can maintain that fetuses have an interest in remaining alive, being healthy, and so forth. But, as we have seen, the (standard, unmodified) sentience view asserts that only sentient beings have interests, potential sentience being insufficient. If this is correct, then a human being's moral status is not determined by kind membership but by a particular property: the (present) capacity to experience feelings. Another view, of course, is that personhood—in the sense requiring an already developed capacity for complex forms of consciousness—is necessary and sufficient for moral status, or perhaps full moral status. So it is far from self-evident that one's moral status is determined by one's essential kind. As far as I can see, the Appeal to Our Essence and Kind Membership lacks any strong grounds for its assumption about the basis of moral status. My sense is that this third important pro-life argument is driven by (1) uncritical acceptance of the idea that personhood is necessary and sufficient for moral status—an idea with roots in the Biblical notion of God creating all nonhuman creatures for disposal by humanity—and (2) conflation of personhood with membership in Homo sapiens. The conflation may be due to the discredited idea that natural kinds are susceptible to classical definitions—in this instance, that humankind can be defined as "rational animal" (see note 35). Whether or not my speculations are correct, the Appeal to Our Essence and Kind Membership cannot be considered sound because it has provided no compelling reason to accept its second premise about the basis of moral status. And again, its assumption that rationality is essential to our species is highly dubious.

DOES THE GOOD SAMARITAN ARGUMENT CLINCH THE CASE?

None of the three strongest pro-life arguments has proved persuasive. This strengthens the case for the earlier-defended framework for understanding prenatal moral status, which can withstand the challenges of these arguments. At this point, with an eye on the abortion issue as opposed to embryo research, I will consider whether the so-called Good Samaritan Argument (GSA) clinches the case for the moral permissibility of abortion in at least a broad range of cases. What is most striking and novel about this argument is that it grants to the pro-life position the seemingly pivotal assumption that the fetus is a "person" in the moral sense: a being with full moral status and a right to life.[36]

So let us assume, for the sake of argument, that the fetus has a right to life in the same sense that you and I do. It may appear to follow from this assumption that abortion is, perhaps with some exceptions, morally impermissible. The GSA, however, contends that abortion is permissible in a wide range of cases (not just a few exceptional ones) even if the fetus has a right to life. Introduced by Judith Thomson, the GSA has recently been developed and refined by David Boonin, whose discussion I take to be representative.[37]

In the renowned thought-experiment, you awake and find yourself in a hospital, hooked up to a violinist who can survive his kidney ailment only if you, who alone have the right blood type, remain in the hospital bed for nine months with the violinist attached to you. He unquestionably has a right to life. To unplug him in less than nine months will guarantee his death. Nevertheless, it seems obvious that you have no obligation to undergo such a great burden to save his life. While being such a good Samaritan would be highly praiseworthy, going to such lengths to assist another person (whom one did not consent to assist) is well beyond the call of duty. Importantly, it is not that your rights to liberty and bodily integrity trump his right to life. Rather, there is no conflict of rights because his right to life does not encompass a right to use your body. The GSA contends that, even if the fetus has a right to life, unwanted pregnancy is relevantly similar to the situation involving you and the violinist. Terminating pregnancy with abortion, like disconnecting the violinist, is permissible.[38]

Is this argument successful? Surely it is permissible to disconnect the violinist, so critics of the GSA must argue that pregnancy and the imagined hospital scenario are dissimilar in at least one morally important respect. I will argue that several considerations—responsibility, the parent-child relationship, and the killing/letting die distinction—are, in combination, sufficient to cast significant doubt on the GSA. I argue not that the GSA fails, but that it is uncertain that it succeeds, except in a small range of cases.

Let us begin by considering the matter of responsibility. In non-rape cases— that is, where a woman has had intercourse voluntarily and becomes pregnant— she (along with the biological father) is responsible for the situation in which the fetus needs life support. Boonin helpfully distinguishes two senses of responsibility: (1) A is responsible for the fact that B exists, and (2) A is responsible for the fact that, given that B exists (anyway), B needs A's help. In the violinist case, you are not responsible in either sense; similarly with pregnancy due to rape. In non-rape cases, a woman is responsible in sense (1)—she helped to create the fetus—but not in sense (2), because the fetus cannot exist independently of the woman's assistance.

Boonin next presents a case in which A is responsible for B's existence in sense (1) in a different way—by extending rather than starting a life—but not in sense (2).[39] Imagine that you, B's physician, saved his life seven years ago in the only possible way: by administering a medication that cured his disease but would predictably cause kidney failure seven years later. Now, as expected, you alone can rescue him from his present ailment by giving him the use of your kidneys for nine months. Surely you are not obliged to accept this burden. You are responsible for B's existence, because you saved him, but not for his neediness given that he exists, since he could not have lived to the present day in a non-needy state. According to Boonin, "where you are responsible in sense (1) and not in sense (2) for the fact that another now stands in need of your assistance . . . the individual in need has not acquired the right to your assistance."[40] Appeals to responsibility, he argues, do not prevail in non-rape cases and, of course, they do not apply in rape cases. They therefore do not refute the GSA.

But let us consider responsibility further, together with the killing/letting die distinction and the parent-child relationship. In discussing the GSA, McMahan helpfully states that "it is very hard to believe that it is permissible to kill one's own child in order to avoid the burden of providing the aid that one has caused it to need."[41] Again, we assume for the sake of argument that the fetus, like a child, has a right to life. And, except for hysterectomy and hysterotomy—rare procedures that pose special risks to the pregnant woman—current methods of abortion involve killing the fetus. By contrast, unplugging the violinist seems to be a case of letting die rather than killing. Moreover, though the pregnant woman is not responsible for the fetus' neediness in sense (2)—it is false that the fetus would have existed even if she had not caused its neediness—she and the biological father have through voluntary action caused the fetus to exist in a needy state, whether or not they conscientiously attempted to avoid this result by using birth control. Let us focus on a sense of responsibility (one compatible with either of Boonin's two senses) that may help us get to the heart of the matter: A is responsible for the fact that B exists in a state in which B needs A's assistance. In non-rape cases, one is responsible in this sense, which arguably grounds a right to assistance—or, more minimally, a right not to be killed—at least when B (who is assumed to have a right to life) is one's own child.

Suppose that you, the physician in Boonin's case, had seven years ago saved the patient, who now, as expected, cannot survive without the use of your kidneys for nine months. Assume that the burden to you is roughly comparable, overall, to the burden of a typical pregnancy in terms of nausea and other discomforts, impact on mobility, and so on: very substantial but less than confinement to bed the entire time. Finally, assume that the patient is your own child. In Boonin's presentation of the case, which indicates no special relationship beyond that of doctor to patient, you do not seem obligated to give the patient use of your kidneys. But you may well have such an obligation if the patient is your child. A fortiori, it is dubious that you may kill your child in order to avoid the burden, comparable to a full-term pregnancy, of providing assistance that you have caused her to need.

But there is an ambiguity in the phrase "your child." It might refer to someone who is socially your child: You are raising him or, if he is grown up, have already raised him. The present challenge to the GSA is strongest if one imagines a parent-child relationship of this sort. But "your child" might refer to someone who is only biologically your child. Perhaps you gave him up for adoption immediately after he was born, or maybe you just furnished gametes for his conception. The biological sense of "your child" seems more applicable in the thought-experiment because, when abortions are sought, a biological mother does not want to become a social mother to the individual in question. But it is not clear that you have any special responsibility at all to someone who is merely your biological child. Let us assume that the individual in question is your biological child, whom you gave up for adoption and with whom you never had any relationship—except for serving as his one-time doctor and saving his life seven years ago. May you let him die in order to avoid a pregnancy-like burden that saving him again would impose on you? I am fairly confident that you may. May you kill him if doing so is the only possible way to avoid this burden (admittedly a very hard circumstance to picture)? It is not at all clear to me that you may. True, you did not want biological parenthood, and you refused social parenthood, but maybe just bringing the kid into the world (even accidentally) through voluntary action is enough to entail that you may not kill him in order to avoid burdens comparable to pregnancy.[42] Here I have in mind burdens that are typical of pregnancy. If the burden would include, say, your death (as with some pregnancies), I would judge that you may, in self-defense, kill the individual, even if he is innocent of any intention to kill you.

Here, therefore, is a reply to the GSA based on appeals to responsibility and one or two further considerations. If allowing one's (merely) biological child to die in order to avoid the burden one has caused her to need is sometimes permissible when killing would not be, as I tend to believe, then this reply to the GSA invokes both the (biological) parent-child relationship and the killing/letting die distinction. If so, it will not apply to methods of abortion that do not involve killing. And, again, there can be no appeal to responsibility in rape cases. So a successful reply to the GSA along these lines would mean that the GSA could justify abortion only in (1) rape cases, (2) any other cases in which a girl or mentally compromised woman is not responsible for being pregnant (as discussed later), (3) cases in which the mother's life is at stake (killing being permissible in self-defense even if the threat is innocent), and, if I'm correct, (4) cases of abortion that do not involve killing. Because these types of cases constitute such a small proportion of abortions,[43] this result would largely defeat what is commonly believed to be a successful argument for the permissibility of abortion.

My cautious conclusion is not that the GSA clearly fails to justify abortion in a wide range of cases, but that there are very substantial reasons to doubt that it succeeds. This suggests that the GSA does not clinch the case for the permissibility of abortion. So I will not rely on the GSA in countering the pro-life position. The tripartite framework, especially the TRIA, remains crucial to my case for the permissibility of abortion.

REASONABLE DOUBTS AND PLURALISM REGARDING PRENATAL MORAL STATUS

On the basis of my tripartite framework and critique of leading pro-life arguments, I have defended the following basic picture of prenatal moral status. First, because sentience is sufficient for having interests and moral status, the sentient fetus has moral status. Again, sentience is likely to emerge no earlier than the beginning of the third trimester (which is later than the vast majority of abortions are sought and, of course, long after embryo research is possible). Whether the sentient fetus has full, or only partial, moral status depends on whether sentience is sufficient for full moral status. Regarding the beginning of our existence, I have somewhat tentatively argued that we originate somewhere between the 16-cell stage and about two weeks of gestation. If so, then the zygote and early embryo (by which I mean an embryo prior to the origination of one of us) has no significant claim to moral status. Such beings have no intrinsic properties such as sentience or complex forms of consciousness that lay claim to moral status. Nor can they develop into—become—such beings because they are not numerically identical to any sentient being or person of the future. What about late (post-origination) embryos and pre-sentient fetuses? I have argued that these human organisms have little or no moral status. The argumentative road therefore may appear smoothly paved for liberal views, and no other views, on abortion and embryo research.

Actually, I think not. I have defended an outline of what I believe to be the most defensible position on prenatal moral status. But I may have erred in some of my reasoning. Or, even if I have not erred—even if I'm right that the position I have outlined is the most defensible—there may be another position or several other positions that are nearly as defensible. I am very confident that the position I have sketched is a reasonable position. I am not confident that no alternative position is reasonable. In fact, I am pretty sure that this is not the case. Unlike nearly every philosopher I know who holds a liberal view on prenatal moral status and/or the ethics of abortion and embryo research, I believe that a broadly pro-life approach remains standing as a reasonable option.

To be sure, there almost certainly will have to be some exceptions to the asserted impermissibility of abortion for the pro-life approach to remain reasonable. For example, based on the plausible claim that one may intentionally kill a person, even an innocent person, as a last resort to save one's own life, I suggest that an exception must be made for cases in which the woman's life is at stake. Moreover, because someone impregnated through rape bears no responsibility for her situation, an abortion in rape cases seems justified—assuming one may kill the violinist, as painlessly as possible, if there is no other safe way to free oneself from him. But a reasonable pro-life view need not admit many exceptions. It might, for example, embrace the conception view of our origination, which would suggest that even zygotes and early embryos have a right to life. Then again, it might not; it might claim a later time for our origination and for that reason prove more permissive about destroying zygotes and early embryos. In any case, I maintain that a broadly pro-life view is a reasonable option.

Let me elaborate on why I think so, notwithstanding my defense of the tripartite framework. Certainly, the biological view of our essence, identity, and origins does not block a pro-life view—which, indeed, presupposes some version of the biological view, even if there is room to quibble about details. Nor does the view that sentience is closely tied to moral status preclude a pro-life view. Nearly all fetuses are potential sentient beings and potential persons. Finding the View that Potential is Sufficient to be about as compelling as the View that Sentience is Necessary, we left open the question of whether having the potential for sentience—or personhood—entailed an interest in surviving so that one could become sentient or realize the life of a person. Such an interest could be the basis of a right to life. For this reason, the TRIA of the harm of death was a crucial part of my framework: Without the TRIA, pre-sentient fetuses could be judged to have full moral status based on their potential (with exceptions, naturally, for those lacking the potential).

Although I believe that the TRIA makes more sense than competing accounts of the harm of death, I also believe there is room for reasonable disagreement on this point. The TRIA is motivated by various intuitions about the comparative magnitude of the harm of death in different cases. These intuitions are not shared by everyone. Even if they were—or should be—shared, perhaps there is a way of accounting for these intuitions that is consistent with a pro-life view. Moreover, the TRIA faces its own challenges. For example, some believe that it has unacceptable implications regarding the ethics of infanticide.[44] At least one scholar has challenged the coherence of the concept of a time-relative interest.[45] Rather than address these and other challenges here, I simply note that there are such challenges and acknowledge that one might responsibly doubt that any version of the TRIA will adequately address them. We have also found reason to doubt that the GSA establishes the moral permissibility of abortion (except in a small range of cases). Such doubts, I submit, leave a broadly pro-life approach standing as a reasonable view about prenatal moral status.

How should we conceptualize this plurality of reasonable views? We might judge that there are several views that it is reasonable to hold only because we have yet to identify an argument or set of arguments that will settle the issue of prenatal moral status once and for all—at least in the minds of adequately informed, reasonable people. This suggests the possibility that some such body of reasoning is "out there" if only we could discover it. If that is the case, then perhaps continued intellectual labor will enable us to identify the correct view as the correct view. On the other hand, even if there is a uniquely correct view and some body of reasoning that could in principle show that this view is uniquely correct, perhaps—due both to our intellectual limitations and to the complexity of the abortion issue—we will never be in a strong position to say, with confidence, that we know that a particular view is the correct one. We may never be in a position to grasp that body of reasoning or, even if we can, we may not be able to ascertain that it is definitive—that it settles the debate. That seems quite possible to me. It would be a problem of moral knowledge.

Another possibility, which I take seriously, is that there is no uniquely correct view on prenatal moral status; rather, there is a range of reasonable views. If so, then no amount of information, insight, logical reasoning, or other resources that can improve our moral thinking could direct us, in practice or in principle, to a uniquely correct position. My taking this metaethical possibility seriously should not be understood to mean that I embrace moral relativism, a view that I find completely implausible. For this metaethical possibility requires no such sweeping denial of the objectivity of ethics. All it requires is the belief that ethics may be partly indeterminate: that there may be some ethical issues on which there is, at the end of the day, a plurality of more or less equally defensible yet incompatible views. A metaphor may help to illuminate this idea of partial indeterminacy in ethics: a hunk of Swiss cheese. Perhaps ethics is objective in the sense of having uniquely correct answers to most ethical questions—picture the solid parts of the cheese—while also having holes of indeterminacy. If so, that would explain why on some issues (abortion, embryo research, perhaps animals' moral status, and/or the finer points of distributive justice) consensus seems especially elusive, without implying, insanely, that there are never correct answers to ethical questions.

FROM MORAL TO POLITICAL PHILOSOPHY: RESPONDING TO REASONABLE PLURALISM

I have argued that there is an impasse, a plurality of reasonable views, on the issue of prenatal moral status. Nor is the range of reasonable views narrow, as they would be if, say, they were all variations on a liberal approach; the range, as we have seen, is very wide. How, then, can we proceed in a discussion of the ethics of abortion and embryo research? My suggestion is first to recall that these ethical issues arise at two levels and then to move our analysis to the level we have yet to address. The ethical issues arise at the level of individual choice (e.g., "Is it morally permissible for this woman in these circumstances to have an abortion?") and at the level of public policy (e.g., "Is it morally defensible for the State to prohibit women from having abortions in these sorts of circumstances?"). Our discussion so far has taken place at the level of individual choice. Insofar as what is right at this level may not translate smoothly into what our laws and other public policies ought to be—for example, there is no law, nor should there be one, against the unethical behavior of speaking rudely to one's relations—we should now ask about defensible public policies regarding abortion and embryo research. I submit that the best policy responses to reasonable pluralism about prenatal moral status will be fairly liberal.

Consider that conservative policies on the issues in question necessarily involve significant government-imposed limitations on liberty—on a woman's liberty with respect to her own body and major life choices if abortion is prohibited or severely restricted, and on the scientific community's freedom of inquiry if embryo research is banned or severely curtailed. Any government, of course, must impose some restrictions on liberty through the mechanism of enforceable law. But, a government appropriately imposes significant restrictions on liberty on the basis of moral values only if there is an overwhelming moral case—at the level of individual morality—for the restrictions.[46] Such is the case in the legal prohibitions of rape, murder, and child abuse. As far as abortion and embryo research go, there is reasonable pluralism and no overwhelming moral case. This warrants some sort of liberal policy response.[47]

Consider the matter this way. For the pro-life view to be correct, several controversial assumptions must all be correct. For the sake of clarity in exposition, I will articulate the most conservative version of the pro-life view, noting along the way that certain amendments or qualifications are possible within a broadly pro-life approach. The first assumption concerns our origins:

1. We human beings come into existence at conception.

This assumption can be modified by replacing the last two words with "within the first two weeks after conception" or the like to reflect an alternative biological understanding of our origins. The second assumption concerns our possession of moral status:

2. We have full moral status, including a right to life, throughout our existence.

From these two premises it follows that we have full moral status, including a right to life, from the moment we come into existence at conception. The third pivotal assumption concerns the relationship between full moral status and the morality of abortion and embryo research:

3. If we have full moral status from the time of conception, then abortion and embryo research are impermissible.

This assumption takes the possession of full moral status to be decisive to the ethics of killing embryos and fetuses. From these three premises, the conservative conclusion follows:

(C) Abortion and embryo research are impermissible.

I have argued that it is reasonable to believe these premises—with the qualification that (3) and therefore (C) need to be modified to permit a few exceptions to the claim of impermissibility. Now I want to emphasize that it is reasonable to disbelieve one or more of these premises. Yet all three must be correct for the conclusion to be well-supported.[48]

The first premise can be reasonably doubted. I have defended a modified version of this premise on the basis of a biological view of our essence and identity; one could accept this modification and remain broadly pro-life. But, as noted earlier, mind essentialism—the view that we are essentially minds—should be regarded as a contender among views of our essence and identity. One might reasonably embrace mind essentialism, which implies that beings of our kind do not originate until sentience emerges in fetal development, sometime in the third trimester. If this is true, then the pro-life view cannot be correct.

As for (2), that we have full moral status throughout our existence, I have defended and deployed the TRIA in challenging this premise. But even one who doubted the TRIA might reasonably doubt (2): It is not self-evidently true, and the major arguments advanced in its favor proved less than compelling. One might reply that, while (2) is not self-evident in a strict sense, it is nevertheless highly plausible. I am sure that many people regard it as highly plausible. Yet many liberals do not—and sometimes even plausible theses can be responsibly rejected on the basis of a countervailing theoretical consideration (e.g., the TRIA) if the latter is sufficiently well supported.

Like the first two premises, the third—that full moral status on the part of fetuses would entail the impermissibility of abortion and embryo research—is also open to reasonable doubt. The GSA constitutes a powerful reason to question (3). Our examination of the GSA raised significant doubts about this argument, but we certainly did not refute it.

The upshot is that the significant deprivations of liberty demanded by a conservative position on abortion and embryo research rest on three debatable
premises. Laws and policies that significantly curtail liberty generally should
not rest on moral positions about which consensus among reasonable people is
so sorely lacking. In effect, women should have the prerogatives of deciding the
contested matter of prenatal moral status for themselves and of making highly
personal decisions regarding whether to have an abortion. Similarly, scientists
should have the prerogative of deciding the moral status of embryos for themselves and pursuing embryo research if they think it appropriate. Whether the
federal government should fund such research, however, raises distinct issues
such as (1) whether partial deference to the pro-life sensibilities of a sizable
portion of the public justifies withholding public funds from embryo research,
and (2) whether such money is well spent on this investment in view of a variety of factors (e.g., alternatives to embryo research, competing claims for
public funds). We will consider such issues in the final section of this chapter.
What is clear at this juncture is that embryo research should not be prohibited.

REFLECTIONS ON THE BASIC SHAPE OF JUSTIFIED POLICIES

Abortion

What would be the general shape of justified policies on abortion? I will take
current American abortion laws as the point of departure for my analysis.

The U.S. Supreme Court's decision in Roe v. Wade (1973) had the effect, for all
practical purposes, of legalizing "abortion on request."[49] According to the
Court, it was unconstitutional for a state to have laws prohibiting the abortion
of a pre-viable fetus—that is, a fetus prior to the time at which fetuses can be
born and kept alive with medical technologies (which, at that time, was around
the end of the second trimester). A woman, the Court contended, has a consti-
tutionally guaranteed right to privacy, on the basis of which she has a right to
terminate a pregnancy prior to viability—although a state, for reasons relating
to its interest in maternal health, may restrict the manner and circumstances in
which abortions are performed after the first trimester. A woman's nonabsolute
right to terminate a pregnancy gives way, or may give way, to the state interest
in fetal life at the point of viability: "For the stage subsequent to viability the
State, in promoting its interest in the potentiality of human life, may, if it
chooses, regulate, and even proscribe, abortion except where it is necessary, in
appropriate medical judgment, for the preservation of the life or health of the
mother."[50]

In its decision in Casey (1992), the Supreme Court did not overturn Roe v.
Wade, as many expected, but reaffirmed its "essential holding" that a woman

has a constitutional right to have an abortion prior to the point of viability.[51] Moreover, the Court preserved *Roe*'s rule that states choosing to regulate or proscribe abortions post-viability must allow exceptions in cases in which the woman's life or health is at risk. However, the Court abandoned the trimester framework of *Roe* in light of medical advances that better protected maternal health and promised to push viability to earlier stages of pregnancy. In a significant development, the Court adopted an "undue burden" framework for determining the constitutionality of certain procedural requirements for obtaining abortions—for example, 24-hour waiting periods and other requirements that are supposed to promote an informed decision by the mother, parental notification requirements, and spousal notification requirements. According to the Court, the informed consent and parental notification provisions in question passed legal muster whereas the requirement of spousal notification did not.

Much of the reasoning and wording of these two decisions have been rightly criticized. For example, the use of the terms "potential life" and "potentiality of human life" is conceptually monstrous. And what is most at issue for women is presumably less a concern of privacy than one of liberty with respect to a woman's own body and life plan. No matter. I will consider whether the basic legal framework established for abortion in the United States is more or less sound as understood from the perspective of justified public policy. Thus, my exploration is not a legal analysis, which would address legal precedents and the content of the Constitution, but a moral analysis at the policy level. Before turning to this analysis, let us note two further components of the legal status quo.

In *Harris v. McRae* (1980), the Supreme Court addressed the constitutionality of the so-called Hyde amendment, which had passed through Congress with strong pro-life support. The Hyde amendment restricted federal Medicaid funding to cases in which the pregnant woman's life is at risk and cases of rape or incest. Upholding this policy, the Court judged that a woman's right to abortion does not encompass a right to have society pay for it.

Another part of the legal status quo concerns the use of a rare, late-term abortion procedure known medically as intact dilation and extraction (intact D & X) and popularly, at least among opponents, as "partial-birth abortions." Sometimes used for late second-trimester abortions and more often for third-trimester abortions, intact D & X, in its most common form, involves the partial, feet-first delivery of a fetus followed by extraction of the brain in order to collapse the skull, so the head can pass through the cervix. In *Stenberg v. Carhart* (2000), the Supreme Court struck down Nebraska's ban on intact D & X for, among other reasons, its ambiguous formulation. Congress later passed the Partial Birth Abortion Ban Act of 2003, which the Court (perhaps reflecting a change in membership) upheld in *Gonzalez v. Carhart* (2007). According to the Court, because intact D & X is not the only possible late-term abortion procedure and is never necessary to protect a woman's life or health, the Partial Birth Abortion Ban Act is not unconstitutional for failing to include such an exception.

Bringing these elements of the legal status quo together, we find this picture:

1. Abortion is entirely permissible prior to viability;
2. States may restrict or prohibit post-viability abortion except where necessary to protect the woman's life or health;
3. Procedural requirements such as parent notification and a 24-hour waiting period are permitted if and only if they do not constitute an undue burden to the pregnant woman;
4. Federal funds will not be spent on the provision of abortions (with a few exceptions);
5. Intact dilation and extraction is prohibited.

Let us briefly consider these elements in turn.

The conjunction of elements (1) and (2) is, I think, very appropriate policy. Its liberality is justified by reasonable pluralism regarding the pre-sentient fetus. The cut-off point of viability, at which time states may set restrictions on abortion, is surely debatable, but I believe it is optimal for public policy purposes. Fetuses are thought to be viable near the end of six months' gestation, which is around the earliest point at which fetuses may become sentient. Sentient beings have moral status; whether or not they have full moral status, the same as a person, is reasonably disputed. Many people believe that a late-term, sentient fetus has full moral status including a right to life. Nearly everyone agrees that a sentient infant has full moral status, and it is probably at least implicit in many people's thinking that a viable fetus could already be a newborn infant and therefore should have the same moral status. In view of these points, and out of respect for the sensibilities of those who are pro-life, I think the viability criterion is optimal. Only if the time of viability moved much earlier in gestation (perhaps a couple of months earlier) would I think that this criterion should be abandoned, in the interest of ensuring that women have ample time in which to secure abortions. Some states may prohibit or substantially restrict post-viability abortions. Requiring exceptions where necessary to protect the woman's life or health is appropriate given a woman's right to self-defense: One may, as a last resort, kill to save one's life or even to protect one from a grave threat to one's health, even if the threat is entirely innocent of bad intent.

As for the third element of the legal status quo, the undue-burdens criterion for procedural requirements also strikes me as reasonable. Although having to wait a day to have an abortion is inconvenient, there can be no denying that the decision is momentous and that time for reflection can help to promote genuinely informed consent (without being unduly burdensome). By contrast, requiring wives to notify their spouses of their decision to abort would be an undue burden due to the likelihood that many women who were pregnant "illicitly" would be subject to spousal abuse.

Turning now to the status quo's fourth element, I, unlike many liberals, believe it is acceptable to prohibit the provision of federal funds for abortion services (preferably with exceptions, as discussed in the next paragraph) so long as that is the choice of duly elected representatives. That women have the right to terminate pregnancy does not mean that the public has to pay for abortion. The pro-life community is a substantial minority of persons whose views are not unreasonable and who have to tolerate very permissive policies on abortion. From the standpoint of their sensibilities, it likely would seem to add insult to moral injury to have to pay for abortions with public funds. To some extent, this sensibility is reflected by acts of Congress such as the Hyde amendment. At the same time, if Congress chooses to abandon this funding restriction based on a different weighing of the values at stake—more emphasis, say, on pluralism and economic justice for the poor—that, too, would be reasonable.

Where a society's duly elected representatives decide to prohibit public funding for abortion, I believe that it would be best to make exceptions in two kinds of cases: where a mother's life or health is at stake and in cases of what I call "no responsibility." Some individuals are not responsible for their pregnancy in the sense that their taking part in an activity (sex) that carried the risk of pregnancy was either involuntary and/or uninformed in a relevant way. Rape victims are obviously not responsible. Nor, in some cases, are minors who are impregnated by other minors if they did not really understand the risks they were taking and, for the purposes of their decision to have sex, not responsible in the way a competent adult would be. The same may be said for some severely mentally impaired adults, who may sometimes have pregnancy-causing sex—perhaps with others who are similarly impaired—without being coerced yet without "knowing what they were doing." So the relevant category justifying an exception is "no responsibility," with rape being one instance. At the same time, I reject incest as a ground for a categorical exception. Probably, most cases of incest that lead to pregnancy involve rape of a minor by an adult family member. But where incestuous sex is voluntary and informed, among adults, I see no special reason why a society should feel compelled to make an exception and fund an abortion (although disgust alone may motivate an exception).

Moving on to the court decision about "partial-birth abortion," my reaction is more critical. Contrary to the law that was upheld, it is not the procedure itself—with its partial delivery of the fetus—that matters. What matters is the stage of fetal development. So a more justified policy would be to permit this procedure in those rare instances when it is performed pre-viability. And, as with post-viability abortion in general, it should be up to states to determine whether to restrict or ban this abortion procedure after the point of viability. So the law about intact D & X is redundant where it is justified and overreaching where it is not. Moreover, the court's claim that the procedure is never necessary for the woman's health is disputed among medical experts and represents an inappropriate intrusion into a pregnant woman's prerogative to defend herself. The Partial Birth Abortion Ban Act was upheld by an irresponsible decision on the part of the Supreme Court.

Embryo Research

The kind of embryo research that has received the most academic and public attention in recent years is embryonic stem-cell research (ESCR). Another type of embryo research that has attracted considerable attention is research cloning (prematurely called "therapeutic cloning" by many proponents). There are other types of embryo research as well, but what is common to all of them—or at least all that are the subject of this discussion—is that the research entails the destruction of embryos.[52] The issues I will consider are (1) whether the research in question should be legally permitted, (2) whether creation of embryos for the purpose of using them in such research should be legally permitted, and (3) whether public funds should be dedicated to the research. The major factors to be taken into consideration in forging justified policy are reasonable pluralism about embryos' moral status, the value of scientific freedom of inquiry, the medical promise of embryo research, the moral sensibilities of the pro-life community, the possibility of viable alternatives to embryo research, and—in connection with the funding issue—alternative ways to use public funds.

Let us begin with ESCR, which is thought to hold the greatest medical promise among the varieties of embryo research. First, some background. A human embryo reaches the blastocyst stage of its development about five days after fertilization. At this stage, the embryo contains an inner cell mass that normally would develop into the fetus and an outer layer of cells that normally would develop into the placenta. The cells of the inner cell mass—embryonic stem cells—can be extracted to develop into virtually any type of human cell or tissue. They are thus described as pluripotent. (By contrast, the cells of an embryo through the eight-cell stage are totipotent—capable of forming a new embryo). Embryonic stem cells are thought to have tremendous therapeutic potential, especially in regenerative medicine, in view of their versatility. It is hoped that ESCR can lead to therapies for many diseases and impairments, including Parkinson's disease, Alzheimer's, diabetes, heart disease, and spinal cord injury, to name just a few. Importantly, deriving stem cells from an embryo at the blastocyst stage requires destruction of the embryo. Due to disagreement over the embryo's moral status, the aspect of embryo destruction generates the most ethical controversy surrounding ESCR.

The legal status quo of ESCR—indeed, of all embryo research—is somewhat up in the air. At the end of the George W. Bush administration, it was roughly the following: (1) Federal law prohibited federal funding of research that involved the destruction of embryos except for studies using embryonic stem cells derived from the small number of cell lines created prior to Bush's August 2001 executive order on the subject, (2) federal law prohibited federal funding for any research that involved the creation of embryos for purposes that would involve their destruction, and (3) there was no significant federal regulation of embryo research conducted in the private sector. President Barack Obama reversed Bush's restriction on federal funding for ESCR and clinical trials were approved, apparently auguring a new era of publicly supported research. However, a federal judge stunned the research community with an August 2010 ruling that Obama's more permissive funding policy actually violated the law against federal funding of research that involves embryo destruction. This decision was reversed in April 2011 by the D.C. Court of Appeals and, at the time of this writing, the legal door has opened to federal funding for ESCR.

As for the issue of morally defensible policy, three factors are paramount: reasonable pluralism about embryos' moral status, the value of scientific freedom of inquiry (which is generally agreed to establish a rebuttable presumption against government interference), and the extraordinary promise of this research. The sensibilities of the minority who oppose ESCR (reasonably) on the basis of their view of embryos' moral status must be taken into account, but how to do so is not obvious. This factor does not justify prohibiting such research. Might it justify a prohibition on public funding? I would argue that it does not—biomedical research being a fundamentally public enterprise—unless and until it is demonstrated that alternatives to ESCR have comparable medical promise.

Some scientists believe that "adult" stem cells (stem cells derived from full-grown human beings) have such promise, meaning there is no medical advantage unique to ESCR. This argument gained momentum in the wake of several breakthroughs in which differentiated "adult" cells were genetically modified into a stem-cell-like state, resulting in induced pluripotent stem (iPS) cells.[53] Much remains uncertain about the potential of iPS cells, however, and it seems very possible that ESCR has unique long-term therapeutic potential, especially in light of some recent findings.[54] The reasonable course at this time, it seems, is to provide substantial public funds both for ESCR and for alternatives—especially iPS cell research—that avoid embryo destruction. If it becomes apparent on the basis of solid scientific evidence that iPS cell research is just as promising as ESCR, then it would be appropriate for our elected government officials to consider withholding public funds from ESCR out of deference to the minority's reasonable sensibilities. Until such a time, the great promise and possibly unique value of ESCR leave no doubt that public money is well invested in this research enterprise.

Is it ethical to create embryos for the express purpose of using them in research that will entail their destruction? According to a prominent school of thought, it is morally preferable to use embryos left over from fertility clinics, which would otherwise be discarded, than to create new ones for research. This thinking is consistent with Obama's executive order, which left in place the prohibition of federal funds for research involving the creation of embryos that would be destroyed. I do not find this reasoning cogent.[55] The embryo's moral status— whether it is full, partial, or no moral status—is the same whether or not the embryo is going to be discarded. If embryos had full moral status (and this were the only reasonable view), then either they should not be produced for fertility purposes, or they should be produced in smaller numbers such that none is ever discarded unless it died of natural causes; accordingly, they should not be sacrificed for medical purposes. Analogously, the fact that someone is terminally ill, or waiting on death row to be executed, does not justify killing him even for important medical purposes; it does not matter that the individual is "going to die anyway." But, in fact, there is reasonable pluralism about embryos' moral status, in view of which it is acceptable to kill embryos for research purposes. It is also acceptable, on account of pluralism, to create embryos for fertility purposes. So it is hard to see why it would not also be acceptable to create them for research purposes.

One might object, however, that to create embryos solely for research purposes is to commodify them. To create embryos for fertility purposes, by contrast, is to afford them a significant chance to be implanted and come to enjoy the life of full-grown human being, which is hardly a way of commodifying them. To allow spare embryos from fertility clinics to be used in research, the argument continues, permits them to be dedicated to a noble research enterprise while avoiding the crassness of creating them for this purpose. But this reasoning makes sense only if we assume that embryos have partial moral status: enough so that concerns about commodification can have a foothold, but not so much that we must prohibit the turning over of spare embryos to research laboratories instead of waiting for them to be "adopted." Thus, this reasoning does not do justice to the plurality of reasonable views that includes the view that embryos lack moral status. Finally, if embryos have only partial moral status, as this reasoning assumes, it is entirely unclear why we should not create embryos in support of the noble enterprise of biomedical research. So the creation of embryos for ESCR, or any other type of embryo research, seems no less justified than the conduct of such research.

Let us finally consider research cloning, which is frequently asserted to promise unique medical opportunities. Stem cells extracted from cloned human embryos, produced specifically for research through somatic cell nuclear transfer—which involves removing the nucleus of a somatic cell, transferring it to an egg whose nucleus has been removed, and stimulating the egg into a state of totipotency—may prove uniquely valuable in studying genetic diseases and developing novel therapies. One major prospect for using cloning to derive embryonic stem cells would be to derive the stem cells used to treat a particular patient from her own cloned somatic cell, thereby avoiding the tissue mismatches that cause immune rejection. (This advantage of avoiding immune rejection has also been claimed on behalf of induced pluripotent stem cells derived from a patient's somatic cells.) Another important possibility would be to clone embryonic stem cells from people with particular diseases to generate a limitless source of cells that can be used to study these diseases without having to extract tissue samples from patients.[56]

Does the fact that the stem cells derive from an embryo produced through cloning make any moral difference? I submit that it does not matter. There is nothing inherently wrong with cloning to produce an embryo. There are special concerns (taken up in Chapter 6) about reproductive cloning, the use of somatic cell nuclear transfer to create an embryo with the intention of implanting it and bringing the fetus to term, but research cloning is not reproductive cloning; and research cloning can be safely and appropriately circumscribed by making it illegal to implant a cloned embryo into a woman's uterus. Research cloning as part of ESCR poses no novel difficulties. It is simply a way of creating embryos for research, which, we found, poses no moral difficulties beyond those involved in embryo research per se.

NOTES

1. I develop this thesis in *Human Identity and Bioethics* (Cambridge: Cambridge University Press, 2005).
2. For an excellent theoretical treatment of narrative identity, see Marya Schechtman, *The Constitution of Selves* (Ithaca, NY: Cornell University Press, 1996).
3. See, e.g., Lynne Rudder Baker, *Persons and Bodies* (Cambridge: Cambridge University Press, 2000).
4. *Human Identity and Bioethics*, chap. 2.
5. This point is powerfully developed in Eric Olson, *The Human Animal* (New York: Oxford University Press, 1997).
6. A version of this view, according to which we are essentially *embodied minds*, is developed in Jeff McMahan, *The Ethics of Killing* (New York: Oxford University Press, 2002), chap. 1.
7. Ibid.

8. I address these challenges in *Human Identity and Bioethics*, chap. 2. For a discussion that perceives the balance of arguments as favoring mind essentialism over the biological view, see McMahan, *The Ethics of Killing*, chap. 1.

9. See, e.g., Patrick Lee, "The Pro-Life Argument from Substantial Identity: A Defence," *Bioethics* 18 (2004): 249–63. Remember that I am using the term "person" to refer to those who are indisputably persons. Pro-life thinkers often use the term to apply to any member of our species from conception on.

10. The discussion that follows draws significantly from my "Moral Status, Human Identity, and Early Embryos: A Critique of the President's Approach," *Journal of Law, Medicine & Ethics* 34 (2006), pp. 50–54.

11. Thanks to Alfonso Gomez-Lobo for making me aware of these competing models.

12. Lee Silver, *Remaking Eden* (New York: Avon, 1997), p. 45.

13. Helen Pearson, "Your Destiny from Day One," *Nature* 418 (July 4, 2002): 14–15.

14. Gregor Damschen, Alfonso Gomez-Lobo, and Dieter Schoenecker, "Sixteen Days? A Reply to B. Smith and B. Brogaard on the Beginning of Human Individuals," *Journal of Medicine and Philosophy* 31 (2006), p. 171. See also Alfonso Gomez-Lobo, "Individuality and Human Beginnings: A Reply to David DeGrazia," *Journal of Law, Medicine & Ethics* 35 (2007): 457–62. Both articles cite S. F. Gilbert, *Developmental Biology*, 6th ed. (Sunderland, MA: Sinauer, 2006) and Pearson, "Your Destiny from Day One."

15. I take it that distinctions of sex and of species are largely biological, partly conventional. By contrast, distinctions of race seem to be largely conventional, partly biological.

16. For an elaboration of these arguments, see my *Taking Animals Seriously: Mental Life and Moral Status* (Cambridge: Cambridge University Press, 1996), pp. 56–61.

17. Another, subtler position would be to hold that infants have the moral status of persons because (1) they have the potential to become persons, and (2) they already have moral status on the basis of another property, viz., sentience. In other words, potential matters if and only if one is sentient, a view that implies that pre-sentient fetuses lack moral status. See Elizabeth Harman, "The Potentiality Problem," *Philosophical Studies* 114 (2003): 173–98. I am skeptical of this view because of the ad hoc way that it connects the importance of sentience and potential.

18. Feelings include not only sensations but also emotions and moods. Thus, an individual who lost all sensory capacity but was still capable of feeling upset, for example, would remain sentient and have interests.

19. See Gary Varner, *In Nature's Interests?* (New York: Oxford University Press, 1998). Cf. Albert Schweitzer, "The Ethic of Reverence for Life," in Tom Regan and Peter Singer (eds.), *Animal Rights and Human Obligations* (Englewood Cliffs, NJ: Prentice-Hall, 1976): 133–38.

20. See, e.g., Joel Feinberg, *Harm to Others* (Oxford: Oxford University Press, 1984); Peter Singer, *Animal Liberation*, 2nd ed. (New York: Avon, 1990); and Bonnie Steinbock, *Life Before Birth* (New York: Oxford University Press, 1992). For my development of this approach, see *Taking Animals Seriously*.

21. For a prominent example of an interests-based account of rights, see Joseph Raz, "On the Nature of Rights," *Mind* 93 (1985): 194–214.

22. See, e.g., Singer, *Animal Liberation* and Steinbock, *Life Before Birth*.

23. See, e.g., Susan Lee et al., "Fetal Pain: A Systematic Multidimensional Review of the Evidence," *JAMA* 294 (2005): 947–54.

24. Strictly speaking, the capacity for consciousness is not equivalent to sentience—the capacity for feelings—because, in principle, a being might be capable of having conscious states such as thoughts but incapable of having feelings. In the world as we know it, however, all creatures capable of having conscious states are sentient.

25. See, e.g., Mary Mahowald, "Respect for Embryos and the Potentiality Argument," *Theoretical Medicine and Bioethics* 25 (2004): 209–14 and Eugene Mills, "The Egg and I: Conception, Identity, and Abortion," *Philosophical Review* 117 (2008): 323–48. For helpful replies to such arguments, see Alfonso Gomez-Lobo, "On Potentiality and Respect for Embryos: A Reply to Mary Mahowald," *Theoretical Medicine and Bioethics* 26 (2005): 105–10 and Gomez-Lobo, "Does Respect for Embryos Entail Respect for Gametes?" *Theoretical Medicine* 25 (2004): 199–208.

26. This theory has roots in Derek Parfit's reasoning about prudential value (*Reasons and Persons* [Oxford: Clarendon, 1984], Part 3) and was explicitly formulated in McMahan, *The Ethics of Killing*. Benefitting from McMahan's ideas, I have developed a version of the TRIA and applied it to issues connected with prenatal moral status (see, e.g., "The Harm of Death, Time-Relative Interests, and Abortion," *Philosophical Forum* 38 [2007]: 57–80).

27. The question of who is harmed more by death must be distinguished from another question: Who is typically better off at the time of death? The second question concerns not only the harm of death but also the amount of good one enjoyed while alive. Clearly, in typical cases the older victims of death have enjoyed more good in life than have younger victims. Thus, one might claim that the 25-year-old who dies is better off, overall, than the infant who dies: The young man is tragically harmed by death but had enjoyed lots of good before that time whereas the infant is substantially harmed by death but had enjoyed almost no good before that time. So one can acknowledge that the young man who dies is better off, overall, than the infant who dies *and* judge that death harms the young man more than the infant. Now, the 10-year-old who dies may seem roughly as badly off as the infant who dies. This coheres with the judgment that, while the child had enjoyed considerably more good than the infant had, death harms the child much more than the infant, making their overall prudential situations comparable.

28. These three factors are enumerated in McMahan, *The Ethics of Killing*, p. 75.

29. His classic article is "Why Abortion is Immoral," *Journal of Philosophy* 86 (1989): 183–202.

30. The discussion in this section draws from my "Must We Have Full Moral Status Throughout Our Existence? A Reply to Alfonso Gomez-Lobo" *Kennedy Institute of Ethics Journal* 17 (2008): 297–310.

31. "Does Respect for Embryos Entail Respect for Gametes," p. 79.

32. This paraphrases an argument presented in Lee, "The Pro-Life Argument from Substantial Identity," p. 250. Essentially the same argument is developed in Christopher Kaczor, *The Ethics of Abortion* (New York: Routledge, 2011), possibly the strongest book-length defense of the pro-life position.

33. "The Pro-Life Argument from Substantial Identity," pp. 252–53.

34. Ibid, p. 262. See also Gomez-Lobo, "On Potentiality and Respect for Embryos: A Reply to Mary Mahowald," p. 109.

35. My sense is that the present argument wrongly attributes to us two distinct essences. I agree that we are essentially human animals, and I can accept (setting aside some doubts) that *human animal* is a natural kind. The problem, in my judgment, is that natural kinds are generally not susceptible to classical definitions. As Saul Kripke has argued, our original concepts for natural kinds typically come by way of ostension: in the case of a species, "this kind of thing" (*Naming and Necessity* [Cambridge, MA: Harvard University Press, 1970]). So a natural kind such as our species would be "defined" by ostension, not by means of a description. Aristotle thought, by contrast, that the human being was both a biological kind and a kind susceptible to classical definition, namely "rational animal." To believe this today, in my opinion, is philosophically naïve and reflects a failure to understand leading contemporary work on natural kinds.

36. Our use of *person*, by contrast, has been purely descriptive—applying to beings that meet a certain description—rather than implying anything about moral status.

37. Judith Jarvis Thomson, "A Defense of Abortion," *Philosophy and Public Affairs* 1 (1971): 47–66 and David Boonin, *A Defense of Abortion* (Cambridge: Cambridge University Press, 2002). Boonin draws not only from Thomson but also significantly from Frances Kamm's work. See especially Kamm, *Creation and Abortion* (New York: Oxford University Press, 1992).

38. See Boonin, *A Defense of Abortion*, pp. 135–39.

39. Ibid, pp. 172–75.

40. Ibid, p. 174.

41. *The Ethics of Killing*, p. 398.

42. I agree with Kamm that intentionally killing an innocent person is sometimes justified, but requires more justification than letting an innocent person die (*Creation and Abortion*, p. 31). Accordingly, in order to justify killing, the burden one would face if the individual is not killed would have to be a lot higher than the burden that would be sufficient to justify allowing to die.

43. By "abortions," I really mean those that involve a medical procedure—what people generally have in mind when using the term. I do not mean to include the use of birth control methods that work (at least sometimes) by preventing implantation of early embryos, thereby allowing them to die. If we included these instances of birth control as abortions, then the category of abortions that do not involve killing would be considerably larger.

44. See, e.g., Matthew Liao, "Time-Relative Interests and Abortion," *Journal of Moral Philosophy* 4 (2007): 242–56. I reply to this charge in "The Harm of Death, Time-Relative Interests, and Abortion," pp. 76–80.

45. Ben Bradley, "The Worst Time to Die," *Ethics* 118 (2008): 291–314.
46. One might think that this principle implies either that infanticide should be legal or that there is an overwhelming moral case against infanticide at the level of individual morality. I disagree, however, because it seems clear to me that prohibiting people from killing infants is not a significant restriction of personal liberty.
47. For a formidable discussion of reasonable pluralism and its political implications, see John Rawls, *Political Liberalism* (New York: Columbia University Press, 1993).
48. I assume that no pro-life argument that did not make these assumptions would be promising. In view of how consistently these assumptions are made by pro-life thinkers, including the academics among them, I consider my assumption fairly safe.
49. United States Supreme Court, *Roe v. Wade*, 410 U.S. 113, 93 S.Ct. 705 (1973).
50. Ibid.
51. *Planned Parenthood of Southeastern Pennsylvania v. Casey, Governor of Pennsylvania*, United States Supreme Court, 112 S. Ct. 2791 (1992).
52. A statistical analysis of data involving embryos, for example, could be considered embryo research, but it would fall outside the present discussion.
53. See Rob Stein, "Scientists Report Advance in Stem Cell Alternative," *Washington Post* (9/26/08): A17 and Rob Stein, "Cell Technique Works Without Embryos," *Washington Post* (10/1/10): A2.
54. Andy Coghlan, "Stem Cell Bust as Mice Reject Own Tissue," *New Scientist* (May 21, 2011): 10.
55. Here I find common cause with Dan Brock, "Creating Embryos for Use in Stem Cell Research," *Journal of Law, Medicine & Ethics* 38 (2010): 229–37.
56. Andy Coghlan, "UK Cloners Target Diabetes Cure," *New Scientist* 183 (August 21, 2004): 8–9.

3

Creation Through Genetic Enhancement

The most straightforward sense in which we create human beings is through reproduction. A looser sense of "creation" is at issue in the present chapter. We sometimes speak of a person's changing so much that she becomes *a new person*. If such major change is pursued self-consciously by the agent, we might say (with a bit of exaggeration) that she is involved in *self-creation*. If genetic technologies of the future permit us to fashion a radically new kind of human being, we may speak more literally of *creating people* or at least of *creating new kinds of people*. These realities and possibilities provoke ethical and philosophical issues.

Human beings have always been interested in self-improvement and the cultivation of their children. We diet, adopt an exercise regimen, change our hair color, and modify habits of work and leisure in efforts to change ourselves in ways that we consider improvements. Many parents teach their children to read and require them to read regularly; society follows up by making them go to school for many years whether they want to or not. Parents may add piano lessons or tennis camp to the regimen. Technologies, many of them familiar, are sometimes involved in such self-improvement and cultivation projects. Pianos, for example, have been around for centuries. Diet pills, exercise machines, and hair dye are not so old, but not particularly new either. Somewhat newer are certain biomedical means of facilitating personal improvement—or *enhancement*, as it is often called in biomedical contexts. Thus, while cosmetic surgery has been around for decades, the ad hoc use of Ritalin by college students and the use of erythropoietin by competitive cyclists are more recent phenomena.

Moreover, various genetic enhancements of our minds and bodies represent possibilities down the temporal road.

This chapter will address ethical issues provoked by the prospect of genetic enhancement. The focus on this mode of enhancement is motivated by its close tie to the concept of creating human beings, or types of human beings, and its tendency to provoke some of the strongest, most interesting moral objections within the debate over enhancement. Moreover, the issues provoked by the prospect of genetic enhancement seem less well understood than the issues raised by presently existing enhancement technologies. In exploring genetic enhancement, the chapter will devote special attention to issues pertaining to *human identity* and *human nature*, both because of their philosophical interest and because these topics tend to be addressed very inadequately in the literature on enhancement. One thing the chapter will *not* do is offer a comprehensive discussion of the ethics of enhancement or even the ethics of genetic enhancement in particular. Rather, it will explore the ethics of genetic enhancement insofar as the latter relates to human identity, human nature, and kindred philosophical themes. Accordingly, the ethical discussion will organize itself around two questions:

1. Is genetic enhancement morally problematic for reasons connected with human identity?
2. Does it pose morally unacceptable threats to human nature—and perhaps, thereby, to humanity?

The sections that follow begin with a brief exploration of the concept of enhancement. Next, they present several examples of possible future genetic enhancements. Eight of these have a fairly clear basis in current scientific understanding and in that sense may be considered nearer-term; two others are far-fetched and have the feel of science fiction, given the current state of technology, but are certainly conceivable—perhaps more conceivable than the Internet was a century ago. The chapter then turns to the concept of human identity in relation to enhancement. Providing the bulk of the ethical analysis, the next two sections develop and address concerns about (1) authenticity (an identity-related value) and (2) perceived risks to human nature (and possibly humanity itself), referring back to the previously described possibilities for genetic enhancement. The overall position defended could be described as fairly liberal.[1]

ON THE CONCEPT OF ENHANCEMENT

As already noted, human beings have long been interested in self-improvement and the cultivation of their children, both of which involve enhancement. Used broadly, the term *enhancement* can be applied to many everyday activities (exercise, musical or athletic training), institutions (education, specialty camps), and products (hair dye, diet pills). In biomedical contexts, enhancements are commonly understood as interventions that are intended to improve human functioning or form beyond what is necessary to restore or maintain health.[2] Stated another way, enhancements are interventions to improve human functioning or form that do not respond to *genuine medical need*, where the latter is defined either (1) in terms of disease, impairment, illness, or the like; or (2) as departures from normal (perhaps species-typical) functioning. Thus, enhancement is commonly contrasted with *treatment* or *therapy*, which responds to genuine medical need. Accordingly, use of exercise, hair dye, surgery, and genetic technologies of the future will count as enhancements when the desire for self- or other-improvement, not medical illness or impairment, motivates the interventions.

Naturally, the concept of enhancement can be illuminated by way of contrast with treatment only if there is a meaningful distinction between the two. This might be doubted in view of such examples as the following. Children who are very short due to a deficiency in growth hormone are classified as receiving treatment in getting synthetic growth hormone. Meanwhile, children who have normal levels of growth hormone, but are equally short simply because their parents are short, count as medically normal, so their receiving synthetic growth hormone counts as enhancement—despite their being equally disadvantaged by short stature and standing to gain in the same way from the drug. Also challenging the treatment/enhancement distinction are certain cases of psychopharmacology. In these cases, patients who have no psychiatric illness or dysfunction use a psychotropic medication in order to feel better in wrestling with their (ordinary) psychological issues and to improve their (already normal) levels of functioning. One might contend that, since such patients struggle with psychological and interpersonal phenomena that can be ameliorated with medication, it means little to say that they are not ill whereas a person who, say, barely qualifies as having depression or general anxiety disorder is ill.

Undoubtedly, the treatment/enhancement distinction will seem arbitrary in a range of cases because our distinction between normal and abnormal health will sometimes seem arbitrary. Notwithstanding the gray area between treatment and enhancement, however, the distinction seems compelling and meaningful in many or most contexts. Many scenarios involving muscle-building, cosmetic surgery, discretionary use of medication, and genetic technologies of the future furnish paradigm instances of enhancement. Moreover, it may be sensible to accept the distinction for the sake of argument even if its conceptual status is debatable. Opponents of biotechnological enhancements generally rely on the distinction in order to identify the class of interventions they oppose. Because I defend a cautious liberalism regarding genetic and other types of enhancement, I prefer to assume the conceptual field on which the debate over their appropriateness most frequently takes place—and then evaluate so-called enhancements on their merits. Hereafter, therefore, I will assume that "treatment" and "enhancement" are meaningful, contrasting terms.

At the same time, it is noteworthy that enhancement can be defined independently of treatment by focusing on the extension or augmentation of *capacities*. Here is one promising definition for the biomedical context: "a biomedical enhancement is a deliberate intervention, applying biomedical science, which aims to improve an existing capacity that most or all normal human beings typically have, or to create a new capacity, by acting directly on the body or brain."[3] Although the word "typically" seems redundant given the reference to most or all human beings, the definition has advantages. First, it does not rely on a contrast with medical treatment, thereby sidestepping the controversy about the treatment/enhancement distinction. That eliminates any need to decide whether or not a candidate enhancement takes one beyond normal functioning or health. Second, it suggests a helpful definition of enhancement in general: An enhancement is a deliberate intervention that aims either to improve a capacity that most or all normal human beings have or to create a new capacity. This nicely covers not only biomedical enhancements but also athletic and musical training, education, and competence with computers. There may be other advantages of this and similar definitions. In any case, for the remainder of the discussion, I will conceptualize enhancement by contrast with treatment when engagement with other commentators or some other practical purpose favors this standard understanding. But most or all of the discussion will be consistent with the definition in terms of capacities as well.

POSSIBLE GENETIC ENHANCEMENTS OF THE FUTURE

We turn now to several possibilities of genetic enhancement, beginning with those that are nearer-term.

HIV/AIDS Immunity

Taking a clue from certain prostitutes who manage to avoid infection with HIV—the virus that causes AIDS—despite engaging in high-risk behaviors over many years, scientists have identified a gene that plays a crucial role in HIV infection. The gene programs the building of a receptor on cells that functions as an entryway for the virus. Those who have two mutated versions of this gene (one from each parent) and therefore lack the receptor are immune to HIV infection. So scientists may be able to create a gene vaccine containing the DNA sequence that disrupts the functioning of the normal genes that produce the crucial cell receptor. The vaccine could be injected into people by way of viruses or other genetic delivery vehicles ("vectors"), artificially conferring immunity to HIV infection. A less successful genetic intervention would confer partial resistance rather than full immunity. In either case, the intervention would *enhance a person's immune capabilities*. This would therefore be an instance of genetic enhancement, suggesting that some enhancements—those directed at *health preservation through prevention of illness*—are likely to be far less controversial than other kinds of biomedical enhancement.[4]

Muscle Development

At least two scientific findings suggest the possibility of genetically enhanced muscularity in people. First, researchers have demonstrated that injecting mice with a virus containing the DNA sequence responsible for producing insulin-like growth factor results in unusually muscular mice whose muscles are exceptionally resistant to the wasting effects of aging.[5] Second, it has been found that genetically modified mice who do not produce myostatin, a growth factor that controls muscle growth, develop enormous muscles.[6] Similar genetic interventions in humans may have similar enhancing effects.

Learning and Memory Enhancement

In 1999, scientists reported that by inserting into mouse embryos a gene that increases production of a protein implicated in learning and memory, they produced mice who learned far more quickly than other mice and better remembered what they learned. However, the modification also apparently made the mice more sensitive to pain, providing a helpful reminder of the risks of genetic interventions. Because the crucial gene and associated protein appear to be present in other mammals, including humans, the research suggests the possibility of genetic learning and memory enhancement in humans.[7]

Cognitive Enhancement More Generally

The abilities to learn and remember what one has learned are hardly the only aspects of intelligence. Other aspects include the ability to perform complex operations in one's head, the ability to reason logically, and creativity. Further aspects of intelligence, on some accounts, include musicality, the possibly related ability to learn new languages, the ability to understand one's own and others' emotional states, the capacity for complex practical reasoning, and even the sort of spatial and kinesthetic awareness that is found to a high degree in many athletes. No matter how we define "intelligence"—and whether we think there is one global trait that deserves this name or several relatively discreet types of cognitive ability—intelligence has some sort of polygenic (multiple-genes) basis. The environment, of course, has an enormous role in enabling and cultivating intelligence, but it is indisputable that genes play a significant role. This fact alone suggests the possibility, in principle, of introducing genetic material with the aim of globally enhancing intelligence or, perhaps more realistically, enhancing particular aspects of intelligence.[8]

Musical Pitch Recognition

The "multiple intelligences" theory counts musicality as one of several types of intelligence.[9] Whatever its relation to intelligence, musicality involves (among other things) the ability to identify—without an external reference point— different pitches and discriminate among them. There is evidence that musicality, or at least pitch recognition, is highly heritable. Studies have indicated, for example, that pitch recognition aggregates in families[10] and, more decisively, that identical twins (who have virtually identical genomes) have more similar abilities of pitch recognition than do fraternal twins (who are genetically related only as siblings).[11] This suggests the possibility, in principle, of genetic interventions to increase a person's pitch recognition.

Reduced Need to Sleep

Researchers have identified a natural timer called the suprachiasmatic nucleus— or circadian clock—in the hypothalamus, a portion of the brain that regulates the autonomic nervous system. This timer regulates various cyclical phenomena, including wakefulness. Animal studies have demonstrated that two genes together cause the production of a protein that resets the circadian clock. If the same proves true in the human case, one could imagine a genetic enhancement involving neurological cell grafting: Genes for an agent that resets the circadian clock would be inserted into cells that could be implanted in the hypothalamus. Perhaps doing so could reduce an individual's need to sleep by several hours.[12]

Sunnier Dispositions

Although dispositions to experience particular moods and emotional states involve highly complicated phenomena, there is some basis for thinking that genetic enhancement along these lines is a future possibility. Recent decades have witnessed the development of psychotropic medications far more effective than what had been available in the past. Most relevantly in the present context,

selective serotonin reuptake inhibitors (SSRIs)—such as Prozac and Lexapro—
have set the pharmacological standard for ameliorating not only depression, for
which they were originally intended, but also anxiety disorders, obsessive-
compulsive and related disorders, and even sexual paraphilias. Moreover,
although hard clinical data are hard to come by, these medicines have long been
thought to benefit "the worried well" in the absence of any psychological disorder. On the basis of his clinical experience, Peter Kramer reported that some of
his patients—including several who could not be diagnosed with a mental
illness—actually experienced favorable personality transformations.[13] Whether
or not Prozac and other SSRIs have the effect of personality enhancement in
some nontrivial proportion of cases (as seems disputable), there is little doubt
that they can help individuals who face ordinary life struggles but have no psychological disorder in their experience of mood and emotion: People on SSRIs
tend to have sunnier dispositions.[14] Considering that these drugs work by allowing more serotonin, a neurotransmitter, to be available to receiving neurons,
perhaps we will be able to identify one or more genes that have a comparable
impact on a person's serotonin activity. If we do, then genetic interventions—
both for therapy and enhancement purposes—will be one large step closer to
realization.

Delayed Aging Process

Everyone ages. This is true not only in the trivial chronological sense—each
year we get a year older—but also in the physiological sense of aging known as
senescence. Senescence involves such familiar phenomena as gradual wrinkling
of the skin, decrease in muscle tone, partial hearing loss, and graying of the
hair. It also involves increased susceptibility to infections, diabetes, high blood
pressure, and heart disease, among other conditions. Senescence is universal if
one ages enough in the chronological sense, but its timing and severity are potentially subject to medical influence. It may become possible, by genetic modifications to sperm, eggs, or early embryos, to allow people to live longer with
significantly delayed and/or less severe senescence—that is, to allow longer,
healthier lives. Why think so? First, there is considerable evidence that, in
humans, not only longevity but also later onset of senescence runs in families,
suggesting a genetic basis. Second, studies indicate that animals deprived of
food (but provided vitamins and minerals) live longer with later senescence
than other animals—and that altering genes apparently related to food metab-
olism can have similar effects.[15] Insofar as we generally think of physiological
aging as a normal process, and therefore not a target for treatment, anti-aging
genetic interventions would count as enhancements on the standard way of
conceptualizing enhancements.[16]

The next two examples of possible genetic enhancements are presented in thought-experiments about the cumulative effects of multiple, coordinated enhancements over many generations. Both are conceivable. If they are to prove technically feasible, it will be in the distant future.

Post-Humans, a New Species of Hominid

Genetic enhancement has been taking place for several hundred years, during which time the human population has gradually divided into two classes.[17] The Naturals are descended from people who were not genetically enhanced, either because they lacked the funds to purchase the enhancements or because they had moral scruples about them. The Enhanced are descended from people who were enhanced in every generation. After the first round of genetic enhancement, with each later generation it was possible to begin with an already-enhanced human genome and enhance it further. As the years passed, scientific advances permitted reprogeneticists to make ever more complex enhancements with hundreds or thousands of additional genes.

Initially, enhancements focused on physical and psychological health—such as improved immunity and better dispositions to moods—but before long such traits as athletic talent, analytical ability, creativity, and musicality became targets, along with longer lifespans and delayed senescence. New enhancements were added to an expanding foundation shared by everyone among the Enhanced. In order to minimize the chance that genetic interventions would interfere with the pre-existing human genome, enhancements involved the placement of genes on an artificial chromosome. As Enhanced individuals tended to lose romantic interest in Naturals, the former generally reproduced only with each other. And because the transmission of particular genes requires the matching of similar ones in reproductive partners, offspring of one of the unusual Natural-Enhanced pairings were unable to inherit the enhancements from the Enhanced parent's artificial chromosome. After the first generation, all Enhanced individuals had 48 chromosomes—23 natural and one artificial chromosome from each parent. Inter-class reproduction, after a time, began to show significantly higher rates of infant mortality and morbidity than *intra*-class reproduction; and many inter-class couples of normal childbearing age proved unable to achieve pregnancy without intensive artificial assistance.

Social tension between the classes became acute. Enhanced and Natural children mostly attended different schools. Among the adults, the Enhanced occupied all significant university positions, nearly every seat in government, and the leading positions in science, industry, and business. During the early generations of genetic enhancement, many Naturals were as wealthy and well-educated as members of the Enhanced, but this changed. Over time, the

Enhanced became the de facto upper class in economic and educational—as well as biological—terms. Meanwhile, the Naturals became a heavy economic burden.

Three centuries later, reproduction between Naturals and the Enhanced almost never occurs—and is considered extremely distasteful among the Enhanced. They regard inter-class sexual relations in the way that twenty-first-century people regarded sex between a middle-aged person and a young teenager, at best, or between a human and an ape, at worst. Sometimes such sexual liaisons occur, despite their illegality, and occasionally pregnancy results. On the extremely rare occasions that such progeny are not aborted in utero and survive to adulthood, they consistently prove infertile. By one criterion for individuating species, the fact that Naturals and Enhanced cannot produce fertile offspring implies that the two populations have become distinct species. This finding is confirmed by other respected criteria for species individuation, given the massive genetic divergence and resulting separation of phenotypes (observable traits) that have gradually occurred in the age of genetic enhancement. Leading biological anthropologists—all, of course, Enhanced—agree that the Naturals, having undergone little genetic change, continue to represent *Homo sapiens* while the Enhanced constitute a new hominid species. The new species is dubbed *Homo maximus* by scientists, but its members are colloquially referred to as "post-humans."

The next thought-experiment represents a distinct way of thinking about where many generations of enhancements could lead. It identifies a new sort of being not by reference to biology—the emergence of a new species—but by reference to a special kind of superiority. In principle, the two thought-experiments could be combined into one, but they need not be.

Post-Persons, a Superior Kind of Moral Agent

It is several centuries into the millennium.[18] Out of the massive human population, a discrete population has evolved—through successive, carefully engineered genetic modifications available to those able and willing to pay for them—and has achieved a considerable number. These beings are in many respects superior to unenhanced people. They typically learn 10–12 human languages, a feat made possible by their retention throughout their lifetimes of the sponge-like capacity that young human children have always had. Their memories, on average, are as capacious as those considered prodigious among the unenhanced population. They have far more extensive self-awareness than ordinary persons, being able to detect with little or no effort the ways in which their biological endowment, early environment (which they remember very clearly), and present environment create myriad dispositions and pressures to think and behave in particular ways. Being far more rational than ordinary people, they are embarrassed to have evolved from a type of creature so susceptible to superstitions, myths, cultural prejudices, ethnic and religious discrimination, unconscious bias in favor of one's own interests, a litany of logical fallacies, and so on. They marvel at the way even the philosophers and scientists among the unenhanced population regularly deceive themselves about their own strengths and weaknesses, their motives, and the likelihood of adhering to resolutions. Bringing together several of these strengths, the post-persons are vastly superior in their moral capacities. First, they are consistently impartial whenever (but only when) impartiality is morally required. Second, because they screen out distracting stimuli and think very quickly, they reach correct moral judgments in conditions of stress no less consistently than they do in leisurely reflection. Third, they suffer from weakness of will so seldom that any member who does so is regarded as having a psychological disorder. Finally, in comparison with ordinary persons, these enhanced humans are enormously adept at envisioning the likely consequences of their choices and identifying the implications of their moral judgments.

The differences between ordinary persons and post-persons are so great that post-persons tend to regard themselves as *different in kind* from persons. Just as persons tend to say (with some exaggeration) that they are rational while animals are irrational, post-persons tend to say that they are appropriately impartial whereas persons are not. Just as persons tend to regard themselves as agents who plan, in contrast to animals who can barely perceive the future, post-persons regard themselves as far-sighted and accurate in perceiving the future, and as deciding wisely on that basis, in contrast to persons, who are poor prognosticators and worse decision makers. Just as persons tend to think of themselves as moral agents who can be held accountable to one another and of animals as simply not making this grade, post-persons regard themselves as *reliable* moral agents in contrast to the unenhanced, *haphazard* moral agents. While post-persons do not have the disdain for persons that persons so frequently have had for animals, considering such disdain just one more form of group prejudice, post-persons are keenly aware of the many differences separating the two populations. Again, they tend to perceive a difference in kind. Despite some reluctance, unenhanced persons do as well.

In later sections, we will refer back to the nearer-term possibilities for genetic enhancement and to the more distant possibilities of post-humans and post-persons.

HUMAN IDENTITY IN RELATION TO ENHANCEMENT

Various moral concerns about biomedical enhancements invoke the concept of human identity. For example, one team of authors focusing on enhancements of mental function states that "[t]he self-transformation that we effect by neurocognitive intervention can be seen as self-actualizing, or as eroding our personal identity."[19] But what sense of identity is at issue when these and similar sentiments are expressed?

The philosophical literature on human identity—or *personal* identity, as it is usually called—is enormous and growing. I believe that most of this literature makes two fundamental errors. The first is a tendency to conflate two distinct senses of identity—numerical identity and narrative identity—that prove to bear on distinct ethical issues. The second error, in my view, is overestimating the strengths of a psychological approach to our numerical identity and underestimating the strengths of a biological approach. I have defended these claims at length elsewhere[20] and provided a preliminary defense of the biological approach in Chapter 2. For present purposes, it will suffice to clarify the distinction between the two senses of human identity and to recapitulate the basic claims of the competing psychological and biological approaches.

The analytic tradition in philosophy has focused on numerical identity: the relationship something has to itself over time in being one and the same entity. An account of numerical identity furnishes criteria for something of a particular kind to continue to exist through change. Thus, a plant may grow, change color, and wilt before going out of existence. A ship may deteriorate and undergo replacement of certain parts while remaining one and the same ship. Similarly, a person undergoes tremendous changes over the years, yet a single person may reflect on all of these changes as having happened *to her*.

What, then, are the persistence conditions of a human person? What changes are so substantial that they entail that the individual dies or ceases to exist? Theories of what is traditionally called personal identity attempt to answer these questions. (I prefer to speak of *human* identity or *our* identity because the term "personal identity" half-suggests either (1) that we are essentially persons [a very dubious claim that was criticized in Chapter 2] or (2) that we seek criteria for our numerical identity *only so long as we are persons* [whereas we seek criteria for our numerical identity, period].)

According to the psychological approach, our numerical identity consists in some sort of psychological continuity. In most psychological theories, the relevant kind of continuity is continuity of experiential contents, or the maintaining of psychological connections, over time.[21] Examples of such psychological connections are having an experience and later remembering it, forming an intention and later acting on it, and the persistence of particular beliefs and desires.

In some psychological theories, by contrast, the relevant type of continuity is continuation of one or more basic psychological capacities, which may survive the loss of memories and other experiential contents.[22] Examples include a basic capacity for reasoning or, even more minimally, the capacity for conscious experience—either of which could survive complete amnesia. For any psychological theorist, permanent loss of the capacity for consciousness—and therefore of any specific kinds of mental states or psychological connections—entails the end of our existence.

By contrast, the biological approach holds that our persistence over time requires not psychological continuity but the continuation of our (biological) life.[23] As discussed in Chapter 2, according to this view, we come into existence early in gestation, whenever a human organism of our kind emerges (depending on the specific theory, as early as conception and as late as two weeks later). Thus, we existed as pre-sentient fetuses and could continue to exist in an irreversible coma or vegetative state. While few would value the prospect of existing without any mental life, the present approach urges us not to confuse the issue of what is valuable in our existence with the metaphysical-conceptual issue of our numerical identity. According to the biological approach, the most plausible conception of our essence views us not as essentially *persons* (in a psychological sense) or *minds* (beings who are at least sentient if not also persons), as suggested by psychological theories, but as essentially *human animals or organisms*.

The debate between the psychological and biological approaches is a debate over our numerical identity. Most people, most of the time, do not think much about their identity in this sense, which in most contexts is taken for granted. People tend to think more often about their *narrative* identity. Identity in this sense involves an individual's self-conception: her implicit autobiography, central values, and identifications with particular people, activities, and roles. It is the sort of identity at issue when someone has an identity crisis.[24] When an adult experiencing a mid-life crisis asks, "Who am I?" he is typically not wondering about his numerical identity. Rather, he is trying to get his bearings on what is most important to him, how he "defines" himself, and what self-image can helpfully navigate him through important life decisions. Narrative identity straightforwardly involves psychology. Therefore, a proponent of the biological approach to numerical identity can grant that that the psychological approach helpfully captures much of what is involved in *narrative* identity because psychological connections over time are essential to developing, maintaining, and refining a sense of oneself as the protagonist of one's life-story.

At this point, one might wonder whether the distinction between the two senses of identity collapses for defenders of the psychological approach. After all, on this approach, psychology is crucial to both types of identity. Yet the issues connected with the two senses of identity are different. The issue of numerical identity concerns criteria that determine whether a being at one time and a being at another time are, despite change, one and the same being. The issue of narrative identity concerns the content of self-conceptions, not persistence over time; one can remain numerically the same individual despite significant changes in narrative identity. Moreover, narrative identity, unlike numerical identity, is radically particular: What is most central and salient in *my* self-conception? A correct answer for you will not be a correct answer for me, yet, whatever our numerical identity consists in, the criteria will be the same for you and me. Unless we bear in mind the numerical identity/narrative identity distinction, our reasoning about human identity can quickly become mired in conceptual confusion—as occurs frequently in discussions of the ethics of enhancement.

Some scholars believe that numerical identity is implicated in concerns about genetic and other kinds of enhancement. For example, after developing a view of our numerical identity (and noting no other sense of identity), Walter Glannon expresses this thesis in the context of genetic therapy:

> [G]ene therapy designed to correct or treat a cognitive or affective disor-
> der would be more likely [than therapy with no direct effects on mental
> life] to alter one's identity. The manipulation of the relevant neurotrans-
> mitters or regions of the brain that generate and support mental life would
> directly affect the very nature of the mental states definitive of personhood
> and personal identity through time.[25]

Glannon applies this reasoning to already existing persons and not only to embryos, fetuses, and newborns (who, in his view and consistent with the usage
we adopted in Chapter 2, are not persons). Presumably, the claim extends to
enhancements that have comparably far-reaching consequences for someone's
mental life.

However, the thesis that enhancing a person's mental characteristics would
result in a numerically distinct person is utterly implausible. If the biological
approach is correct, as I believe, the thesis is obviously false because a single
human organism survives such improvements of mental life. More importantly,
the thesis is indefensible on *any* contending theory of identity. For starters, the
post-enhancement person will remember his own life prior to the intervention.
(There is no special reason to think that his memory experiences are delusional
in being about *his*, and not *someone else's*, earlier experiences.) Furthermore,
most of his intentions and attitudes are likely to survive the intervention,
though some may change—as they may in any of us. So, even if for the sake of
argument we grant Glannon's dubious assumption that we are essentially persons,[26] there's no reason to believe that enhancing an existing person's cognitive

and affective abilities would disrupt numerical identity. While the psychological approach conceptualizes our identity in terms of mental life, the criterion
for identity is persistence of one and the same mental life—understood either
in terms of psychological connections such as memories or in terms of continuing basic capacities—not persistence of a mental life *with the same specific
abilities and traits*. We might reconstruct Glannon's reasoning this way: He intuitively appreciates that a significant improvement in mental characteristics
can affect *narrative* identity, the person's self-conception; but, failing to distinguish the two senses of identity, he fallaciously applies this intuition to numerical identity, generating a view that implies that one of us is eliminated any time
a substantial psychological enhancement occurs.

   Genetic enhancements, if successful, are likely to affect one's narrative identity
by affecting one's self-conception. Anyone acquiring a much stronger memory,
perfect pitch, or a sunnier disposition will probably perceive herself differently
than she would have in the absence of the change. Are genetic enhancements
or other types of enhancements morally problematic for this reason? Many
commentators and laypersons think so. As I understand their identity-related
concerns, they are best understood as advancing a charge of inauthenticity.

THE CHARGE OF INAUTHENTICITY

Conflating the Two Senses of Identity

Echoing themes developed by McIntyre and Taylor, Carl Elliott has been near
the forefront of commentators expressing concerns about enhancement in relation to authenticity.[27] (These concerns are directed at one's use of enhancement
to change oneself, not parents' use of enhancements to change their children.)
Elliott examines two competing ideals in American culture: (1) self-creation—
deliberate self-development and self-transformation—with few if any moral
constraints on what we can become, and (2) authenticity, which may imply
some constraints. Conceptualizing authenticity as *being true to oneself*, he
explores these two ideals in depth.

   What is the concern about enhancement in relation to authenticity? According to Elliot,

   [w]hat is worrying about so-called "enhancement technologies" may not
   be the prospect of improvement [I should hope not!—Ed.] but the more
   basic fact of altering oneself, of changing capacities and characteristics
   fundamental to one's identity. . . . [Deep] questions seem to be at issue
   when we talk about changing a person's identity, the very core of what the
   person is. Making him smarter, giving him a different personality or even

giving him a new face—these things cut much closer to the bone. . . . They mean, in some sense, transforming him into a new person.[28]

The President's Council on Bioethics expresses a similar worry: "In seeking by these [biotechnologies] to be better than we are or to like ourselves better than we do, we risk 'turning into someone else,' confounding the identity we have acquired through natural gift cultivated by genuinely lived experiences. . . ."[29] The concern, apparently, is that enhancement technologies threaten to alter the self and one's identity in a fundamental way, making one "a new person"—and that such a change is inauthentic.

Once again, it is important to stress that the sense of identity at issue is narrative identity. If genetic enhancement gave you a sunnier outlook than you had before, *you* would change. It is not the case that you would literally be destroyed and another person created in your spatiotemporal wake, as would be the case if numerical identity were disrupted. So, given that it is narrative identity that is at issue, what exactly is the basis for concern?

Much of the worry about creating "a new person" may derive, once again, from conflating the two senses of identity. Consider this reasoning:

1. Enhancement technology X would alter a person's identity.
2. Altering a person's identity is morally problematic.
Ergo
3. Enhancement technology X would be morally problematic.

The charge that a particular enhancement technology would be morally problematic can be understood as asserting that it would be morally problematic for society to make it available, that it would be morally problematic to avail oneself of it if it is available, or both. To say that something is morally problematic is not to say that it is morally indefensible, all things considered, but that it tends to be wrong. In philosophers' terminology, it is pro tanto wrong.

On one natural reading of the argument, it is clearly fallacious. Premise (1) is true only if it appeals to narrative identity. Meanwhile, (2) is safely assumed only if it appeals to numerical identity (ending someone's existence would be a momentous matter). Equivocating on the term "identity" invalidates the inference to the conclusion stated in (3).

On an alternative reading of the argument, however, the argument does not equivocate because identity is construed in the narrative sense in both premises. But then why accept the second premise? What is wrong with a technology that alters someone's narrative identity or self-conception? What would be wrong, or even pro tanto wrong, with her using this technology if she autonomously seeks the change in question? The strongest answer to these questions appeals directly to the concept of authenticity in advancing a charge of inauthenticity.

Narrative Identity, Authenticity, and Self-Regarding Choice

In considering the present objection, recall that authenticity is conceptualized as *being true to oneself*. So, underlying the charge of inauthenticity is the idea that there is some entity—the self—to which one fails to be true, or faithful, in pursuing genetic or another kind of enhancement. This suggests that the nature or character of the self is significantly independent of one's will; otherwise, an autonomous choice to change oneself in a particular way could not involve a failure to respect, or be true to, the self. Thus, the self, according to the charge of inauthenticity, is largely "given," an objective reality to which one's efforts at self-change and other life choices ought to conform.

Although I have no theory of the nature of the self to offer, I suggest that the objection's assumed model of the self is highly misleading. It is more resonant with current understandings of the self to believe that we can change and, to some extent, invent ourselves—that is, our selves—suggesting that the self is not so "given." And however the self is best conceptualized, I will argue, self-transformation through genetic enhancement is not per se an inauthentic act that involves a failure to be true to the self. My claim is supported by further consideration of authenticity and narrative identity.

Whereas the critique under consideration understands authenticity as being true to oneself, I suggest a slightly more expansive understanding: *being true to oneself and presenting oneself to others as one truly is.*[30] Authentic people express who they are through their decisions and actions, without pretense or artifice. Because there is little tension between who they really are and the personas they present to themselves and others, they may strike us as particularly natural and comfortable with themselves. Modifying the shorter analysis of authenticity by adding the idea of presenting oneself truly to others is motivated by the idea that inauthenticity sometimes involves presenting oneself falsely to others.

In college I knew a guy named Caruso who wore a Star of David on his neck chain. This would not be interesting except for the fact that he was not Jewish and had no intention of converting to Judaism. "Jewish chicks love it," he said, referring to the pendant. Now, if Caruso wore the Star of David in order to express his respect for or solidarity with the Jewish people, with no intention of deceiving anyone about his religion, there would be no basis for charging him with inauthenticity. But if, as he seemed to imply, he wore it with the intention of deceiving Jewish women who did not know him very well into falling for him (or into bed with him), his comportment clearly involved inauthenticity (among other things). The inauthenticity would have involved a false presentation of himself, specifically his religious identification, to others. Now, perhaps false presentation of oneself to others can be analyzed as a particular way of being untrue to oneself, in accordance with the shorter analysis of authenticity: being true to oneself. While leaving that conceptual possibility open, I prefer to be explicit in stating that authenticity requires presenting oneself to others as one truly is.[31] Hence my expanded analysis.

The moral wrong in the case just considered involves intentional deception of others. Attempting to deceive others is, of course, pro tanto wrong and the character trait of dishonesty is a moral vice. So part of the explanation of why inauthenticity is morally problematic is that it frequently involves dishonesty towards others.

But inauthenticity can also involve self-deception. Imagine a college student who is socially without pretense, yet lies to himself in an important way. He persistently tells himself that he is a scientific genius—because he wants to believe this—despite massive evidence to the contrary. He presents a false self to himself. He even organizes his life around this self-deception, taking as many science courses as he can (getting Cs and Bs), researching top graduate programs in theoretical physics, and so on. A graduate program desperate for tuition-paying students accepts him. As the years roll on, he continues to organize his inner story around the thesis that he is an underappreciated genius whose weak public performances, such as mediocre grades and later a failure to secure external funding, are all misleading for one reason or another. Here we have a case of inauthenticity that involves no attempt to deceive other people. Instead it involves self-deception, which I take to be a species of failure to be true to oneself. Whether one believes that self-deception involves moral wrong-doing is likely to depend on whether one believes that the person who self-deceives can be expected to catch himself in the folly and desist (a complicated psychological issue that I set aside).

With these two examples of inauthenticity in view, we might wonder whether all cases of inauthenticity involve deception of others or oneself—that is, some form of dishonesty. I think not. Reflection suggests that inauthenticity sometimes involves a failure of autonomy. Consider a young woman who aspires to be a successful movie actress or musician. She has ability, but the competition is fierce and there are few opportunities for a professional breakthrough. Advisors suggest that she improve her rather ordinary physical appearance. They suggest that she dye her hair blonde, diet drastically, and undergo breast-augmentation surgery. That would make her more striking-looking and marketable, they say. The young woman resents the expectation that she conform to sexist norms of female appearance and initially rejects the advice. After a year without professional breakthroughs, and several unsuccessful efforts to find employment outside of the entertainment business, she relents and accepts the advice given earlier. Under pressure, that is, she gives in and sells out.

Intuitively, it seems that her choice manifests a type of inauthenticity, but it need not involve any dishonesty. After the physical transformation, she really is thin and large-breasted, and her hair is now blonde; she does not claim or imply that she is thin without dieting, large-breasted without surgery, or blonde without hair coloring. Nor does she deceive herself. Rather, it seems to me, the inauthenticity consists in a failure of autonomy.[32] She decides on her self-transformation not because she feels good about doing so and not because doing so reflects her deepest values; she makes her decision under great pressure from a culture whose norms of feminine beauty she finds alienating and demeaning to women. She compromises because she sees doing so as the least bad option in a situation that is itself morally compromised. In this sense, the choice does not really flow from who she is and is not true to who she is. Is the inauthenticity of her choice morally problematic? Reasonable people may disagree about whether her choice, given her circumstances, is ultimately defensible. On the other hand, the inauthenticity it involves is certainly morally problematic from a broader societal perspective insofar as it reflects social circumstances that undermine the woman's autonomy. Her self-transformation is inauthentic for being nonautonomous and reflects a morally problematic social environment.

The examples we have considered locate instances of inauthenticity in dishonesty to others, dishonesty to oneself, or a failure of autonomy. I suggest, somewhat tentatively, that self-creation projects that are both honest and (sufficiently) autonomous are ipso facto authentic. What I can assert with greater confidence is this: Even if authentic self-creation requires more than honesty and autonomy—perhaps the satisfaction of a distinct condition pertaining to self-respect—self-creation through genetic enhancement can be perfectly authentic. Any number of examples comes to mind. An athlete may seek genetic enhancement in order to become more muscular and better at her sport. A history scholar may seek genetic enhancement in order to improve her memory with obvious benefits to her work. An aspiring politician may embrace a genetic means to a sunnier disposition. We could multiply examples and add details as needed. The important point is that there is absolutely no reason to assume, in advance, that such cases necessarily involve dishonesty, a failure of autonomy, or the violation of any further requirement for authenticity. There is therefore no reason to assume that seeking self-improvement of one form or another through genetic enhancement is per se inauthentic. Provided details of particular cases, of course, we may sometimes find self-creation projects involving genetic enhancement to be inauthentic, but there is nothing inherently inauthentic about self-creation through these means.

We can make the same point in terms of narrative identity. Use of genetic enhancement is likely to have a significant effect on one's narrative identity, but this effect on identity is not, by itself, morally problematic. After all, what is narrative identity all about? It is about one's self-conception, what an individual considers most important to who she is, her self-told inner story. And who a person is concerns what sort of person she intends to become just as much as it concerns who she has been up to the present. The inner story is ongoing and, to the extent that circumstances permit her to act and live autonomously, she is the author of that story. Indeed, it may be fruitful to think of self-creation very roughly as *the autonomous writing of self-narratives*. To the extent that we self-create or transform ourselves deliberately, thereby affecting (and reflecting) our narrative identity, we express our values and priorities. If we do so in a way that meets the criteria for authentic self-creation, then we act with authenticity. There is no reason to think that this is impossible with genetic enhancement. So, at the end of the day, the charge of inauthenticity proves groundless.

CONCERNS ABOUT THREATS TO HUMAN NATURE

What if changes sought through genetic enhancement were so extensive that they threatened human nature—and possibly, thereby, humanity itself? This would provoke a distinct set of concerns that engage the ethics of genetic enhancement from a societal perspective. Let us give the floor to several authors who voice objections of this kind.

The Concerns

In a well-known book, Francis Fukuyama considers the possible consequences not only of genetic enhancement but of biotechnology in general.[33] Fukuyama argues that genetic engineering, neuropharmacology, and related developments threaten to alter human nature—the basis of our shared sense of human dignity—which in turn, he claims, is the foundation for human rights. Expressing a similar concern with hotter rhetoric, George Annas asserts that inheritable genetic interventions would be "crimes against humanity" and calls for a "human species protection treaty."[34] Like Fukuyama, Annas believes that human nature is the basis of human rights. In a coauthored article, he and colleagues contend that reproductive cloning and inheritable genetic interventions "can alter the essence of humanity itself (and thus threaten to change the foundation of human rights) by taking human evolution into our own hands and directing it toward the development of a new species. . . ."[35] A moment's reflection reveals that reproductive cloning would have *no* chance—and therefore less chance than natural reproduction—of leading to a new species, so we will ignore the preposterous claim about cloning and focus on genetic enhancement. Regarding the latter, the authors worry about the possible emergence of post-humans who, being very different from us humans, might become victims of slavery or genocide or, believing themselves superior, may perpetuate these crimes against humanity.[36] Meanwhile, Jürgen Habermas refers to "the identity of the species" and "the ethical self-understanding of the species" in developing his concerns about genetic technologies.[37] Paramount among his concerns is that use of these technologies, especially genetic enhancements, will threaten moral equality, human dignity, and human rights.[38]

These and like-minded critics believe that genetic enhancement would threaten to cross the boundaries of, or even change, human nature in some way that is morally unacceptable. The basic reasoning behind this view can be unpacked as follows:

1. There is such a thing as human nature.
2. Genetic enhancement threatens it.
3. Threatening human nature is morally unacceptable.

Ergo

4. Genetic enhancement is morally unacceptable.

In evaluating this reasoning, it will be helpful to distinguish two sorts of perceived threats. One is the threat of *surpassing*—crossing the boundaries of— human nature. Doing so may be thought to be either intrinsically wrong or wrong on consequentialist grounds. Another perceived threat is that of *altering* human nature, which, too, may be thought to be wrong either intrinsically or on consequentialist grounds.

Is There Such a Thing as Human Nature?

Some doubt there is such a thing as human nature. Post-modern thinkers, for example, tend to distrust any sort of "essentializing" and believe that to talk of a human nature is to commit this intellectual faux pas. This distrust, however, overreaches, for some things do have essences: Squares are essentially four-sided, gold is essentially a metal, and cats are essentially mammals. Or so it seems to me. At the very least, we must acknowledge that there are powerful theoretical and intuitive grounds for maintaining that certain kinds of things have essential features.[39] Arguably, humanity has essential features, which might be collectable under the idea of a human nature.

Some thinkers believe that an essential human nature underlies our (allegedly) unique moral status. Yet the characteristic features of humanity that we most prize and regard as distinctive are *not* universally possessed by members of our species.[40] Not all members of our species are rational, linguistically competent, self-aware in various ways, morally capable, and so on. While most who lack these traits at a given time at least have them potentially—as with fetuses and infants—some, due to injury, genetic defect, or advanced dementia, do not. There is not a single characteristic that might plausibly be regarded as a basis for special moral status that is universally possessed by human beings. There are some properties that all human beings have, such as being embodied or being descended from lower primates, but these do not distinguish us as persons or as bearers of special moral status. Does this justify skepticism about human nature?

It does not. The mistake is to assume that human nature must involve *essential* features. An essential feature for a kind of thing is a feature that X (e.g., a particular person) *necessarily* has in order to be a member of that kind (e.g., humanity). Fukuyama makes the error of construing human nature in terms of essential features: "What the demand for equality of recognition implies is that when we strip all of a person's contingent and accidental characteristics away, there remains some *essential* human quality underneath that is worthy of a certain minimal level of respect—call it Factor X."[41] We should not be surprised that he never states exactly what Factor X consists in because, again, there is no human quality that is *both* universal among human beings *and* distinctive of the species in a morally relevant way. Fukuyama is on steadier ground when he allows (contrary to his own essentialist claims) that there can be exceptional humans who lack particular characteristics of human nature. In this more sensible tenor, he defines human nature as "the sum of the behavior and characteristics that are typical of the human species, arising from genetics rather than environmental factors."[42]

Before identifying candidates for traits that comprise human nature, let us consider a more developed definition presented by Allen Buchanan:

> Human nature is a set of characteristics (1) that (at least) most individuals who are uncontroversially regarded as mature human beings have; (2) that are recalcitrant to being expunged or significantly altered by education, training, and indoctrination; (3) that play a significant role in explanations of widespread human behavior and in explanations of differences between humans and other animals.[43]

This definition focuses on characteristics that are very widespread, but not necessarily universal, in our species, and that feature importantly in explaining human behavior and distinguishing humans from other animals. It is a very good definition.

What, then, does human nature consist in? A promising strategy for answering this question, I suggest, is to identify features of personhood. After all, our contemporary concept of a person seems to derive from our understanding of what a normal, sufficiently developed human being is like. Accordingly, I suggest that human nature includes such traits as the capacity to act autonomously, a high degree of sociability, self-awareness of various kinds, rationality, moral agency, and linguistic competence.[44] Insofar as human beings are also finite, fallible beings who are not to be confused with deities, I would add the following traits to our sketch of human nature: a tendency toward certain forms of irrationality, tendencies toward aggression and toward hostility to "outsiders," and mortality. (No doubt one could add other traits.) Human nature is the nature of the highly imperfect persons with whom we are familiar. Perhaps, then, we should amend Buchanan's definition by adding the words "and between humans and deities" at the end.

Does Genetic Enhancement Threaten Human Nature?

Returning to the argument just reconstructed, the first premise, that there is such a thing as human nature, is in good standing. The second premise is that genetic enhancement threatens (to change or surpass) human nature. I dissent in part and concur in part.

As for my dissent, let us return to the nearer-term possibilities for genetic enhancement that we considered earlier: HIV/AIDS immunity, muscle development, learning and memory enhancement, cognitive enhancement more generally, musical pitch recognition, reduced need to sleep, sunnier dispositions, and a delayed aging process. If we imagine someone who undergoes all of these enhancements, we imagine a person who has immunity to developing AIDS, who becomes more muscular than she otherwise would have been, who learns faster and remembers more than she would have without the enhancement, and so forth. This all seems perfectly human. There is nothing in this description that would take the individual outside of the current range of human capacities. Some people already have (without enhancement) HIV/AIDS immunity. Some people have perfect pitch. Some people live longer than others without many of the effects of senescence; some people live to 110 years. And so on.

Even if we supposed that an enhancement *extended* the human range, rather than relocating a particular individual within it, that need not involve any surpassing of human nature. We set new standards all the time. Someone who became a little more muscular though genetic engineering than any human had been before would not surpass or change human nature any more than Barry Bonds did when, allegedly using steroids, he set a new home-run record. The same point applies if, through genetic enhancement, someone were able to live for 135 years.

There is already great variation in the human population, and *Homo sapiens*, like any other species, is characterized by a constantly, if very slowly, changing gene pool as a result of spontaneous genetic mutations, changes in environment, particular acts of reproduction, and other familiar phenomena.[45] So what would it take to surpass or change human nature? I suggest two criteria for surpassing human nature and an additional criterion for changing human nature.

First, *the change has to be drastic.* Michael Phelps' world records in swimming represent the fastest human swimming on the planet, but even his greatest performances are similar in kind to what other world-class swimmers can do; they do not transform him, or our species, into an aquatic mammal. To surpass or modify human nature, the change in question must be so extensive that it yields individuals who seem different in kind from the rest of us. A genetic intervention that conferred the capacity to breathe underwater without special equipment might qualify. An enhancement that made people immune to *all* diseases or enabled them to live thousands of years might as well. A second criterion is closely related to the first: *The change in question must transcend human-typical limits in ways that matter substantially to us.* A genetic intervention (or mutation) that gave people two extra digits on each hand and foot probably would probably not matter enough to count as surpassing or changing human nature. By contrast, a cognitive enhancement that enabled someone to remember every post-natal experience he ever had might qualify. Third, in order for a case of surpassing human nature to count as a case of altering it, *the relevant change would have to occur in most members of our species or in most members of a population that was geographically or socially isolated from the rest of humanity.* A few freakishly enhanced human beings would not change human nature even if they surpassed it.[46]

To pose a threat to human nature, enhancements would have to surpass or alter it. Let us assume that the emergence—through genetic enhancement—of a new species, or of a type of being that seemed different in kind from us in ways that matter, would count as surpassing and changing human nature. It is time to return to our two futuristic scenarios.

The enhanced post-humans are a new species, *Homo maximus*, whose qualitative difference from *Homo sapiens* is vast. In the other scenario, the post-persons are distinguished as a new kind of moral agent. Bringing together several cognitive and psychological strengths, they are vastly superior to unenhanced people in their moral capacities. Indeed, they perceive themselves ("reliable moral agents") as different in kind from unenhanced persons ("haphazard moral agents"), much as the latter traditionally viewed themselves in relation to nonhuman animals. In view of the two futuristic scenarios, I concur with the premise that genetic enhancements pose a threat to human nature. Successive genetic enhancements over generations that yielded such beings as these post-humans and post-persons would surpass and alter human nature.

Is it Wrong to Threaten Human Nature?

The final premise of the argument reconstructed earlier is that threatening human nature is morally unacceptable. This premise can be elaborated in more than one way. It might be claimed that threatening human nature is *inherently* wrong—wrong, that is, simply in virtue of the kind of act it is. Alternatively, one might claim that threatening human nature is excessively risky in consequentialist terms. More specifically, one might assert unacceptable danger to humanity, to the genetically modified individuals, or to both. Since we are considering very extensive genetic enhancements, let us shelve the worry about danger to the post-humans or post-persons, who presumably will be able to take care of themselves. Our consequentialist concern is danger to unenhanced humanity.

THE CLAIM OF INHERENT WRONG

Would it be inherently wrong to change or surpass human nature? It is hard to see why it would be. Species are constantly changing, and the changes sometimes result in new species. Species do not have eternal, immutable essences—much less fixed essences *that are to be regarded as sacred*.[47] Suppose, however absurdly, that we could genetically enhance cats, without risking any harm to any cats along the way, so that they enjoyed life more and suffered no ill effects of their new feline existence. This would be a new kind of cat, but that fact alone seems morally irrelevant. Likely harm and benefit, by contrast, seem entirely relevant. Accordingly, I assume that there is nothing *inherently* wrong with "playing God" in the sense of controlling the evolution of particular lifeforms, including our species, rather than leaving their evolution to chance.[48]

CONSEQUENTIALIST CONCERNS

Returning to the claim that changing or surpassing human nature poses unacceptable risk to humanity, we can distinguish two main concerns: (1) that altering human nature by creating a new species would undermine the basis of human rights; and (2) that post-humans or post-persons may pose a threat to unenhanced humanity either because (a) they perceive unenhanced humanity as having a lower moral status, or (b) they can overpower us.

The first concern, that creating a new species of post-humans would undermine the basis of human rights, is wrongheaded. It assumes that the basis of our human rights is our species membership. However common this belief may be, it makes little sense. The term "human rights," which came in favor as the term "natural rights" went out, enjoyed the advantage that it could be deployed against those who would ascribe rights only to certain parts of the human population—white people, say, or men or landowners. In this context, "human rights" helpfully implied that being human was sufficient for having certain basic rights. But even this was not quite accurate insofar as most people deploying the term did not believe that literally every member of *Homo sapiens*— including fetuses, infants, and the severely brain-damaged—had these basic rights. A better term, perhaps, would have been "*personal* rights," which one has in virtue of being a person.[49] Insofar as moral progress has led to the recognition of moral status for sentient non-persons (human and nonhuman) as well as persons, one might hold that the basis of our fundamental rights is our sentient nature rather than our human nature. (In Chapter 2, I defended a sentience view of moral status while leaving open the possibility that personhood conferred full moral status.) In any case, it is not membership in our species that underlies these rights. Even if it were, creating post-humans would not make the unenhanced lose their rights, for they would still be *Homo sapiens*!

The other major consequentialist concern is that that genetic enhancements over time could produce beings who pose a threat to unenhanced humanity either because they perceive unenhanced humanity as having a lower moral status (a moral possibility if the perception is correct) or simply because they can dominate us (an amoral or immoral possibility).

Suppose, first, that enhancements over many generations yielded post-persons who questioned the moral status of the unenhanced. Given their excellence in moral agency, post-persons would not doubt that the unenhanced *have* moral status; as sentient beings and persons, they obviously do. But it might seem to post-persons that their own vast superiority in moral agency grounds a higher level of moral status. Those who think so, let us say, endorse the following hierarchy: (1) Post-persons, as reliable moral agents, have full moral status, which confers rights in the strong sense of near-inviolability (rights that can be overridden only in "supreme emergency" cases); (2) Persons, as haphazard moral agents, have moral status and rights in a weaker sense that demands equal consideration of their interests, but makes them subject to consequentialist trade-offs (as envisioned by act-utilitarianism). The post-persons who accept this view maintain that it gives persons their due. Those who reject this vision believe it represents an unjustified hierarchy. Suppose that proponents of the view prevail and that its implications are carried out. This would mean that persons are sometimes used—for example, as unwilling subjects of risky biomedical experiments—when their use maximizes expected utility. What should we say about this possibility?

From a moral standpoint, I am not sure. My own unenhanced moral capabilities leave me uncertain as to whether the post-persons are correct in claiming a higher moral status. The way they would treat mere persons like me is no worse than act-utilitarianism has always advocated. Yet, for most of us, this is a somewhat frightening prospect. That does not mean it would be wrong, though. If one group of beings really does have higher moral status than another group of beings, then it *is* justified for the first group to use the second group, at least within the limits of equal consideration of interests (as enshrined in utilitarianism).

From a prudential standpoint, however, matters are clearer: *The possible emergence of post-persons entails some significant risk to unenhanced humanity.* If post-persons thought they had higher moral status and were right about this, their limited use of unenhanced humanity would be morally defensible but nevertheless disadvantageous to us. Our moral status would be respected, but we would sometimes be subject to sacrifice in the name of promoting the overall good of society. This would make us less secure than we are in our current situation in which no beings with higher moral status than ours share the planet with us.

There is a much more decisive reason, however, for regarding the possible emergence of post-persons as posing a significant risk: Whatever the truth about comparative moral status, post-persons might behave immorally. True, in view of their greatly superior moral capacities, they are less likely than currently existing persons to make errors in moral reasoning. So long as they are well motivated and attempt to act justifiably, they are highly likely to do so. But what if they are not well-motivated? *Moral agency, of any type or level, is a set of capacities—which comes with no guarantee of appropriate use.* So the greatest threat associated with post-persons falls under the immoral possibility of abuse by beings more powerful than unenhanced humanity. This is also the greatest threat posed by post-humans, who may or may not act morally toward their hominid cousins.

One might reply that, in the case of post-persons, it is highly implausible to think that beings with such remarkable moral capacities would choose to act immorally by mistreating unenhanced humans. Why would reliable moral agents act this way? They would know such behavior is wrong, so they would not engage in it out of moral ignorance. They suffer from weakness of will so rarely that those who succumb to immoral temptation are regarded as mentally ill. Given their moral strengths, what would account for such behavior?

One possible reason is that weakness of will, even if rare, would not be eradicated. Moreover, even reliable moral agents (assuming they are not gods) are capable of misunderstanding what is right, so we cannot assume that they would have to do what they know to be wrong in order to wrong us; they might do the wrong thing while believing it is justified. Further, we must consider the distinct possibility that *quasi*-post-persons—beings who stand somewhere along the path between us and post-persons—may be considerably less reliable in their moral agency than later post-persons. That would make quasi-post-persons more liable to act immorally and quite capable of treating unenhanced persons as tools for their own ends. Finally, we have to remember

that post-*humans*—a new species of hominid—might emerge after generations of accumulated genetic enhancements, and we cannot assume that *Homo
maximus* would be much more reliable in their moral agency than we are. All
told, then, there are substantial consequentialist grounds for concern.

Responding to the Leading Consequentialist Concern:
A Distant Possible Threat to Humanity

In response to this possible threat in the distant future, we must decide what
degree of caution and control is justified. Let us distinguish and evaluate three
approaches, which we may call *Precautionary Prohibition*, *Precautionary Noninheritability*, and *Moderate Regulation*.

According to Precautionary Prohibition, we should embrace a radically conservative precautionary principle according to which *any* risk of great harm to
humanity is unacceptable, and judge accordingly that we should *ban* genetic
enhancement from the get-go. This way, no process that might lead to a dreadful
outcome can get underway. When we concentrate on the fearful long-term possibility of unenhanced humans being dominated and exploited by more powerful beings, Precautionary Prohibition may seem the wisest course. But various
considerations recommend strongly against it.

First, Precautionary Prohibition overshoots in the direction of caution. It
would prohibit the development of any technology that could *possibly*, in the
very distant future, lead to some sort of disaster. Consider the implications. This
approach would require shutting down the fields of robotics and artificial intelligence, which could eventually lead to artificial lifeforms that could dominate and
exploit us. It would require us to discontinue the new field of nanotechnology,
which could possibly lead to some sort of environmental disaster. In the past,
following this approach would have prohibited the development of ships and
airplanes, which massively increased the destructive potential of warfare while
making global pandemics from infectious diseases a far more realistic possibility.
In the twentieth century, Precautionary Prohibition would have shut down the
field of nuclear physics, which, after all, made nuclear annihilation possible.[50] I
take it that these practical implications are absurd and that Precautionary Prohibition would impose an unacceptable straightjacket on scientific innovation.

A second and closely related problem with Precautionary Prohibition is that
it regards the possibility of a calamity as all that matters, setting aside prospects
for benefit as if they were irrelevant. To ignore benefits is irrational. Imagine
that at the appropriate moments in human history there had been careful, societal deliberation about whether to develop ships and airplanes (as opposed to
allowing them to develop, as actually occurred, with little foresight or planning),
with open-minded, realistic consideration of the pros and cons including risks.
What would sensible persons have thought, at the appropriate times, about the

possibility of developing these modes of transportation? One possibility is that they would have judged that the overall prospect for benefits overwhelmed the prospects for harm: Humanity was likely to be much better off, overall and in the long run, for being able to travel across the ocean and through the sky. Another possibility is that they would have judged that they were unable to speculate with much confidence about the balance of possible benefits and risks of these technologies, but that given what was known and what was not known, it would be appropriate to develop these technologies and keep a close eye on them. By contrast, it would have been unreasonable for them to judge on the basis of some long-term risk to humanity that the development of ships and airplanes should be permanently prohibited. I suggest that, with genetic enhancement, we should take a similar attitude about possible benefits and risks. We may reasonably judge either that (1) likely benefits exceed the risks, assuming we take appropriate, feasible measures to contain the risks, or (2) it is very difficult to speculate with much confidence about the benefits and risks, but given what we know and do not know, it is appropriate to proceed cautiously with genetic enhancement. Even if we take the second approach, which I find appropriately modest about our ability to predict consequences, we should not simply ignore possible benefits as irrelevant. They should be borne in mind no less than the possibility of a serious threat to humanity in the distant future.

With that in mind, recall that possible, nearer-term benefits of genetic enhancement include health-related ones such as improved immunity to HIV infection and delayed senescence. Few would deny the great value of such breakthroughs. In the longer term, as Allen Buchanan notes in his distinctive contribution to this discussion, improvements in various cognitive and psychological capacities could have great benefits in the form of higher efficiency in the workplace, which in turn could yield substantial economic benefits to society at large.[51] Buchanan also notes that enhancements may be necessary, or at least extremely beneficial and desirable, as a means of counteracting some of the harmful effects of human culture itself:

> In order to cope with some of the environmental problems our cultural evolution has produced, it may be necessary, among other strategies, to employ biomedical enhancements—perhaps to improve the body's capacity for thermal regulation under conditions of global warming, or to alter skin cells so that they have greater resistance to skin cancer if they ozone layer further depletes, or to sustain fertility if environmental toxins drastically lower sperm counts.[52]

Such enhancements might include genetic enhancements. In the very long term, the sorts of cognitive and psychological enhancements that could lead to improvements in moral agency might prove extremely valuable. Consider how many problems for individual human beings, particular groups, and humanity at large result in significant measure from irrational prejudices, deficits in sympathy and compassion, and other all-too-human shortcomings. To put it another way, enhancement in the direction of—and possibly including—the emergence of post-persons would have many benefits (as well as some risks, as just considered). Morally superior beings might even treat us haphazard moral agents better than we treat each other.

Of course, it is very difficult to predict what enhancements might come about in the very long term and virtually impossible to assign probabilities to possible benefits. But the same is true of risks such as domination by an enhanced group. The crucial point is that we should not fixate on risks without considering possible benefits. From this perspective, Precautionary Prohibition— which would recommend an immediate ban of genetic enhancement—is an unattractive option.

A third difficulty with Precautionary Prohibition is that for entirely practical reasons it may be unworkable. Suppose genetic enhancement is banned in the United States and the European Union. It might be permitted, either explicitly or de facto through the absence of any prohibition, in other jurisdictions. Thus, while the risk of catastrophe might be reduced, it would not be eliminated unless all countries, or at least all of those possessing sufficient resources to develop genetic enhancements, banned this technology. But even a global ban would not entirely eliminate the relevant risks. A black market of genetic enhancements might emerge. Perhaps more realistically, genetic enhancements might emerge in the guise of permitted genetic therapies. For example, the same genetic interventions that provide therapy for those suffering from muscular dystrophy could confer enhanced muscularity in healthy individuals. The same genetic interventions that provide treatment for patients with Alzheimer's disease would confer enhanced memory powers in individuals who have no memory impairment. The very interventions that provide genetic therapy for those with a predisposition to depression could confer sunnier dispositions on those of normal mental health. And so on. Rightly or wrongly, such "off label" uses of genetic therapies will probably be the direction of many advances in genetic enhancement.

For the reasons just enumerated, I reject Precautionary Prohibition, which would ban genetic enhancement from the outset. A respectable alternative is Precautionary Noninheritability: the proposal that we permit the development of genetic enhancements, with appropriate regulation, but prohibit those that are inheritable. Thus, any genetic enhancement would affect only the individual on whom it is conferred; it would not be passed on to future generations. A chief motivation of this approach would be to prevent the emergence of such beings as post-persons and post-humans by way of genetic enhancements that are inherited and accumulated over many generations—without forgoing all the benefits of genetic enhancement. A chief disadvantage of Precautionary Noninheritability is the enormous inefficiency of having to confer genetic enhancements on members of each generation rather than allowing descendants of the enhanced to inherit the advantages their parents acquired through genetic intervention. HIV immunity, for example, would have to be genetically conferred over and over rather than once in a given family line. Another disadvantage is that this approach would not allow genetic enhancements to build on one another from generation to generation, a restriction that would drastically slow whatever progress would be possible and attainable more quickly through inherited, accumulated enhancements. While I find these disadvantages to represent great costs of prohibiting inheritable genetic enhancements, I expect that many thoughtful people will not share this sense of missed opportunities. Precautionary Noninheritability, which takes the benefits of genetic enhancement more seriously than Precautionary Prohibition does, should be considered a contender.

Let me now introduce what I believe to be the most sensible approach for responding to the risks of genetic enhancement: Moderate Regulation. This approach has three components. First, and perhaps obviously, we must maintain strong political institutions that protect individuals and communities with effective domestic and international laws—laws that prohibit slavery, forcible participation in research, and more generally the unjustified exploitation of the weak by the strong—as well as the willingness and resources to enforce then. If effectively maintained, these laws and institutions will prevent unlawful and unjustified domination by a powerful group. Second, there should be enough government oversight of genetic technologies as they accrue over time to provide every reasonable assurance that genetically enhanced people will not prove to be amoral or, worse, immoral by nature. But, as noted earlier, even moral agents can choose to behave immorally. If a sizable group of enhanced individuals became enormously more powerful than the unenhanced, they might choose to dominate and exploit their weaker cousins. Maybe they would even change the institutions and laws that furnish the protection identified earlier in the first point. Humanity therefore has a legitimate security-based interest in preventing enhanced individuals from becoming exceedingly advantaged or powerful *in comparison with unenhanced human beings*. Hence a third feature of the recommended approach: Government oversight of genetic enhancement must prevent enhancements from creating a dangerously large gulf between genetic haves and have-nots.

How might prevention of a dangerously large gulf be effected? One part of the answer would be to make genetic enhancements, or at least some of them, publicly available through a universal health-care system—or, since biomedical enhancements are generally thought to lie outside the boundaries of health care, a universal "biomedical provision" system. (Although it is beyond the purposes of this chapter to address the well-known problem of distributive justice, it is noteworthy that the present suggestion would be a central component to an adequate response to this problem as it concerns genetic enhancements.) But, for any number of reasons, some individuals are likely to decline to use genetic enhancements or to approve their use for their offspring, so the public availability of this technology cannot entirely solve the problem. Therefore, I also recommend an approach we may call *Contingent Future Noninheritability* (really a sub-approach within the approach of Moderate Regulation). If and when it is believed that the gulf between the genetic haves and have-nots is approaching a dangerous level, a policy shift will occur such that only the individual recipient of the enhancement in question—say, superior memory—would acquire the relevant trait; his or her offspring would not. This would prevent the gap between the genetic haves and the have-nots who refuse to undergo genetic enhancement from continuing to grow. Yet it would also permit parents to give a round of (noninheritable) enhancements to their children if they choose. This solution would prevent the feared scenario of group domination while maximally allowing the benefits of genetic enhancement.

CONCLUSION

After providing background on the concept of enhancement, possible genetic enhancements of the future, and the connections between biomedical enhancements and the two senses of human identity, this chapter has endeavored to address two philosophically rich questions that are, for the most part, poorly addressed in the literature: (1) Is genetic enhancement morally problematic for reasons connected with human identity? (2) Does it pose morally unacceptable threats to human nature—and perhaps, thereby, to humanity itself? Now we can summarize our answers to these questions.

The answer to the first question is No. As we found, much of the semi-articulate hand wringing about enhancements' effects on human identity appears to be motivated by a conflation of numerical and narrative identity. On another reading of (some of) the relevant worries, however, there is no conflation because only narrative identity is at issue. This concern resolves into a concern about the authenticity of enhancement through genetic (and other biomedical) means. Our exploration of authenticity, though, neutralized the concern by finding that genetic enhancement could be a perfectly authentic means to self-creation.

The second question concerned perceived threats to human nature and possibly, thereby, to humanity itself. Our analysis of human nature found that there is nothing inherently objectionable about altering or surpassing human nature, something that accumulated genetic enhancements over many generations might actually do. Nor would doing so undermine the basis of human rights. The most legitimate concern was that the long-term effects of accumulated genetic enhancements might include the emergence of beings who were in a position to exploit, dominate, or abuse unenhanced human beings. We found that this long-term possibility did not justify banning genetic enhancements before they got underway, and it probably did not justify limiting them from the outset to those that cannot be inherited. Rather, I argued, the most justified approach, all things (including possible benefits) considered, is Moderate Regulation, one component of which should be Contingent Future Noninheritability, a ban on *further* inheritable genetic enhancements in the event that the gap between genetic haves and have-nots appears close to being dangerously large.

The arguments developed in this chapter have not shown that genetic enhancement is, all things considered, morally justified because our inquiry has been confined to concerns that pertain to human identity or human nature. I happen to believe that genetic enhancement is, all things considered, morally justified, and should be permitted by our laws and policies. But here I can only refer readers to other writings that help to make the case.[53]

It is worth emphasizing that to say that genetic enhancement is morally defensible, and should be permitted by our laws and policies, is not at all to say that it should go unregulated. I have endorsed Moderate Regulation, not *Laissez Faire*. The federal government has a legitimate role in regulating genetic technologies; in the United States, it is currently playing this role in connection with attempted genetic therapies. Such oversight is needed to protect the public welfare. We saw that it would be important to ensure that our enhanced descendents do not become amoral or immoral by nature. It would be at least as important, as just discussed, to make sure that uneven distribution of genetic enhancements does not permit one group within the population to become dangerously more powerful than the rest of the population. And, of course, it would be essential to ensure that genetic enhancements are not made available until research has demonstrated that they are reasonably safe and likely to benefit their recipients.

NOTES

1. In parts of this chapter, I draw in bits and pieces from my "Enhancement Technologies and Human Identity," *Journal of Medicine and Philosophy* 30 (2005): 261–83.

2. See Eric Juengst, "What Does *Enhancement* Mean?" in Erik Parens (ed.), *Enhancing Human Traits* (Washington, DC: Georgetown University Press, 1998): 25–43.

3. Allen Buchanan, *Beyond Humanity?* (Oxford: Oxford University Press, 2011), p. 23.

4. Some commentators classify this sort of intervention as neither treatment nor enhancement, but *prevention* (see, e.g., Erik Parens, "Is Better Always Good? The Enhancement Project," in Parens, *Enhancing Human Traits*, p. 5). This conceptual proposal allows critics of enhancement to avoid the implausibility of opposing such seemingly innocuous biomedical interventions.

5. H. Lee Sweeney, "Gene Doping," *Scientific American* (July 2004): 63–69.

6. Se-Jin Lee, "Regulation of Muscle Mass by Myostatin," *Annual Review of Cell and Developmental Biology* 20 (2004): 61–86. Both types of genetic muscle enhancement are discussed in Julian Savulescu, "The Human Prejudice and the Moral Status of Enhanced Beings: What Do We Owe the Gods?" in Savulescu and Nick Bostrom (eds.), *Human Enhancement* (Oxford: Oxford University Press, 2009), p. 213.

7. Ya-Ping Tang et al., "Genetic Enhancement of Learning and Memory in Mice," *Nature* 401 (September 2, 1999): 63–69. This research is helpfully discussed in Ronald Green, *Babies by Design* (New Haven, CN: Yale University Press, 2007), pp. 77–78.

8. For a good discussion, see Nicholas Agar, *Liberal Eugenics* (Oxford: Blackwell, 2004), pp. 27–31.

9. See Howard Gardner, *Frames of Mind: The Theory of Multiple Intelligences* (New York: Basic Books, 1983).

10. Siamak Baharloo et al., "Familial Aggregation of Absolute Pitch," *American Journal of Human Genetics* 67 (2000): 755–58.

11. Dennis Drayna et al., "Genetic Correlates of Musical Pitch Recognition in Humans," *Science* 291 (March 9, 2001): 1969–72.

12. See LeRoy Walters and Julia Gage Palmer, *The Ethics of Gene Therapy* (New York: Oxford University Press, 1997), pp. 102–3.

13. Peter Kramer, *Listening to Prozac* (New York: Penguin, 1993).

14. For thoughtful reflections on this finding, see President's Council on Bioethics, *Beyond Therapy* (Washington, DC: PCB, 2003), pp. 240–51.

15. I have benefited from an overview of the science in Green, *Babies by Design*, pp. 75–77.

16. For a contrary view, see Arthur Caplan, "Death as an Unnatural Process," *EMBO Reports* 6 (2005 special issue): S72–S75.

17. This is my adaptation of a thought-experiment presented in Lee Silver, *Remaking Eden* (New York: Avon, 1997), pp. 281–93.

18. This is a slightly modified version of a thought-experiment presented in my "Genetic Enhancements, Post-persons, and Moral Status: A Reply to Buchanan," *Journal of Medical Ethics* 38 (2012) (forthcoming).

19. Martha Farah et al., "Neurocognitive Enhancement: What Can We Do and What Should We Do?" *Nature Reviews Neuroscience* 5 (May 1, 2004):421-25.

20. *Human Identity and Bioethics* (Cambridge: Cambridge University Press, 2005), chaps. 2 and 3.

21. Two of the most influential works are John Locke, *An Essay Concerning Human Understanding*, 2nd ed. (1694), Bk. II and Derek Parfit, *Reasons and Persons* (Oxford: Clarendon, 1984), Part III.

22. See, e.g., Lynne Rudder Baker, *Persons and Bodies* (Cambridge: Cambridge University Press, 2000) and Jeff McMahan, *The Ethics of Killing* (New York: Oxford University Press, 2002), chap. 1.

23. The most influential work representing this approach is probably Eric Olson, *The Human Animal* (New York: Oxford University Press, 1997).

24. See Marya Schechtman, *The Constitution of Selves* (Ithaca, NY: Cornell University Press, 1996).

25. Walter Glannon, *Genes and Future People* (Boulder, CO: Westview, 2001), pp. 81–82.

26. Ibid., p. 25.

27. See Alasdair McIntyre, *After Virtue*, 2nd ed. (Notre Dame, IN: University of Notre Dame Press, 1984); Charles Taylor, *The Ethics of Authenticity* (Cambridge, MA: Harvard University Press, 1992); and Carl Elliott, *A Philosophical Disease* (New York: Routledge, 1999) and *Better Than Well* (New York: Norton, 2003).

28. *A Philosophical Disease*, pp. 28–29.

29. *Beyond Therapy*, p. 300.

30. For a more detailed discussion of authenticity and its relationship to narrative identity and self-creation than is presented here, see my *Human Identity and Bioethics*, pp. 106–13. For further reflections on the self in relation to these concepts, see my "Prozac, Enhancement, and Self-Creation," *Hastings Center Report* 30 (March–April 2000): 34–40.

31. It might be slightly more accurate to say that authenticity requires presenting oneself to others as *one thinks* one truly is. Honest mistakes about how one truly is are possible. For example, one might present oneself to others as Italian-American, reasonably believing that one is on the basis of available evidence, though one is actually Greek-American. Hereafter I will ignore this complication, although I will take up cases of self-deception in which there is ample evidence to support a correct self-understanding.

32. I develop and defend a particular analysis of autonomy in *Human Identity and Bioethics*, pp. 95–106.

33. Francis Fukuyama, *Our Posthuman Future* (New York: Picador, 2002).

34. George Annas, *American Bioethics* (Oxford: Oxford University Press, 2005), p. 41.

35. George Annas, Lori Andrews, and Rosario Isasi, "Protecting the Endangered Human: Toward an International Treaty Prohibiting Cloning and Inheritable Alterations," *American Journal of Law and Medicine* 28 (2–3): 151–78.

36. Ibid, pp. 161–62.

37. *The Future of Human Nature* (Cambridge: Polity, 2003). For an excellent discussion of Habermas' concerns, see Elizabeth Fenton, "Liberal Eugenics and

Human Nature: Against Habermas," *Hastings Center Report* 36 (November–December 2006): 35–42.

38. Somewhat similarly, though without the emphasis on human nature, Michael Sandel develops concerns about people's sense of solidarity with one another and their willingness to "stand together" amid great differences in ability and fortune (*The Case Against Perfection* [Cambridge, MA: Harvard University Press, 2007]). For an excellent response to Sandel, see Frances Kamm, "What Is and Is Not Wrong with Enhancement?" in Savulescu and Bostrom, *Human Enhacement*: 91–130.

39. See, especially, Saul Kripke, *Naming and Necessity* (Cambridge, MA: Harvard University Press, 1980).

40. Let us assume, with the authors we have been considering, that the relevant sense of "human" is *Homo sapiens.* "Human" could equally well refer to the full range of hominid species, in which case a new one emerging via genetic enhancement would probably also be human.

41. *Our Posthuman Future*, p. 149, my emphasis.

42. Ibid, p. 130.

43. *Beyond Humanity?*, p. 118.

44. The claim is not that each trait is strictly necessary for personhood. Rather, these properties and perhaps others form a cluster such that a person is a being with *enough* of these properties. Not surprisingly, given this cluster-concept analysis, personhood proves to be a vague concept with blurred boundaries. For a fuller discussion, see my "On the Question of Personhood beyond *Homo sapiens*," in Peter Singer (ed.), *In Defense of Animals* (Oxford: Blackwell, 2006): 40–53.

45. In the human case, there is also cultural evolution on top of biological evolution. Cultural evolution has long affected which human traits endure through the generations. For example, without the inventions of clothing and controlled fire, the whole species might well be hairier.

46. Cf. Norman Daniels, "Can Anyone Really be Talking About Ethically Modifying Human Nature?" in Savulescu and Bostrom, *Human Enhancement*, pp. 25–42.

47. I get the sense that many people who instinctively oppose the intentional alteration of species remain in the grip of Aristotelean biology. Our ethics of genetic enhancement should instead take into account the facts of evolutionary biology.

48. Readers who have doubts about my assumption and would like a more detailed rebuttal to the charge of inherent wrong will benefit from Buchanan, *Beyond Humanity?*, chap. 4.

49. For an outstanding exploration of the concept and basis of human rights, see James Griffin, *On Human Rights* (Oxford: Oxford University Press, 2008).

50. The points about nuclear annihilation and global pandemics come from Buchanan, *Beyond Humanity?*, p. 55.

51. *Beyond Humanity?*, chap. 2

52. Ibid, p. 163.

53. I strongly recommend Green, *Babies by Design* and Buchanan, *Beyond Humanity?* I argue for the all-things-considered moral defensibility of genetic and other biomedical enhancements in *Human Identity and Bioethics*, chap. 6, although I now consider that discussion significantly incomplete. I also recommend Fukuyama, *Our Posthuman Future* and Sandel, *The Case Against Perfection*, which oppose genetic and (for the most part) other forms of biomedical enhancement.

4

Prenatal Genetic Interventions

In Chapter 3 we examined the ethics of genetic enhancement in relation to human identity and human nature. Much of the discussion focused on adults making decisions for themselves. In this chapter, we will consider decisions on behalf of children-to-be: decisions about whether to perform certain interventions on gametes (sperm and egg cells), embryos, or fetuses. These decisions pertain not only to enhancements but to other genetic interventions as well. More specifically, the chapter will consider prenatal genetic diagnosis (PGD), prenatal genetic therapy (PGT), and prenatal genetic enhancement (PGE).

One of the most exciting areas of science today lies at the intersection of assisted reproduction, human genetics, and embryo research. In this burgeoning field of reprogenetics, the human capacity to control the traits of offspring is rapidly expanding. With reproduction, we create human beings. With reprogenetics, we have the potential to create human beings with particular desired traits or without certain undesired traits—that is, to create certain *kinds* of human beings. This creative potential provokes a host of ethical issues. Before turning to those issues, let us briefly consider the status quo of reprogenetics and recall the conclusions about prenatal moral status that were reached in Chapter 2.

BACKGROUND

How close are we to creating genetically modified human beings?[1] At the moment, we can only *select* for or against certain traits. We have been doing this, in fact, for many years—through the genetic analysis of fetal cells obtained from amniotic fluid by *amniocentesis* in the second trimester of pregnancy, and through the genetic analysis of *chorionic villus samples* obtained from the placenta during the first trimester. Given the availability of abortion during the first two trimesters, these techniques have enabled women to decide whether to terminate pregnancies upon receiving positive test results for such disorders as Down syndrome and spina bifida. Thus, these fetal tests have permitted *negative selection*, or selection *against* children-to-be with certain genetic characteristics. Insofar as amniocentesis and chorionic villus sampling (CVS) also reveal the fetus' gender, they have, in principle and sometimes in practice, permitted either negative selection or *positive selection* (selection *for*) on the basis of gender.

Since the mid-1990s, a more powerful genetic technique has come into play. In contrast to the tests just described, which are performed on fetuses in utero, *pre-implantation genetic diagnosis* is conducted on embryos in vitro. Following in vitro fertilization (IVF), which is now commonly employed in the context of assisted reproduction, a blastomere (cell) of an embryo is biopsied—typically at the six- to eight-cell stage, sometimes later—and genetically analyzed. Since IVF can be used to generate several embryos simultaneously, genetic analysis enables prospective parents to select against embryos with identified genetic defects and for embryos that are free of these defects. At the time of this writing, geneticists have identified more than 2,000 disease-related gene mutations for which tests are clinically available.[2] Among the many examples are mutations for cystic fibrosis, Turner syndrome, Alzheimer's disease, X-linked mental retardation, hemophilia, and Lesch-Nyhan syndrome.

Most, but not all, of the conditions presently tested for with PGD are genetic disorders. Another condition—or, rather, trait—that is tested for is gender, as with the older fetal tests. In another use of PGD that is no less controversial than gender selection, embryos have been selected on the basis of their potential to become compatible tissue donors for older siblings who need transplants to address medical conditions. In these cases, a child is created (at least partly) as a means to helping a sibling, provoking ethical concerns about using human beings as mere means for others' benefit.

There are also methods for testing gametes prior to fertilization. As an alternative to embryonic PGD, clinicians can perform similar tests on a woman's ovum—egg cell—by analyzing DNA from the polar bodies (nucleus-containing structures that are shed by the maturing ovum). This type of test is limited, naturally, to the maternal contribution to a potential child's genome. Another type of gamete screening is sperm sorting: the sorting of sperm into those bearing the X chromosome (making them female-producing) and those with the Y chromosome (male-producing). Sperm sorting enables selection by gender.

Every technique we have considered thus far involves prenatal genetic testing and the selection against or for particular traits. Current research, however, is beginning to pave the way for the more radical prospect of prenatally *altering* genomes. One possibility would apply to humans a technique that has been used with mice. The technique begins with the extraction of stem cells from a sufficiently developed embryo (see Chapter 2 for background on embryonic stem cells). Geneticists can then apply *homologous recombination*—a technique using a cell's own gene repair mechanisms to make site-specific changes—to alter the stem cell's genetic sequence in order to eliminate predisposition to a particular disease.[3] Stem cells that take up the desired change can be injected into the original embryo or another embryo derived from gametes of the same parents. A child produced by this approach would be *chimeric*: Some of its cells would contain the desired gene while some would contain the undesired gene. But even this mixing could greatly benefit someone with a predisposition to a recessive disorder—such as cystic fibrosis—in which the disease results from a nonfunctioning gene and the resultant absence of a needed protein. A baby born with a fair number of cells producing the needed protein might be much healthier than a baby born without any such cells.

This chimera-producing approach is unlikely to be successful in connection with diseases caused not by the absence of some helpful gene but by the presence of a dominant, harmful gene. An example is the gene for Huntington's disease, which involves devastating neurological degeneration that begins in middle age. An individual who was chimeric with respect to the gene for Huntington's would be vulnerable to developing the disorder. An alternative approach that could sidestep this difficulty would involve the highly controversial element of reproductive cloning (an issue taken up in Chapter 5). Starting with stem cells derived from an embryo produced in vitro with the parents' gametes, the genetic defect could be repaired in accordance with the technique just described. But, in the present approach, a corrected stem cell could be cloned: With an appropriate chemical or a small electric shock, the stem cell could be introduced into one of the mother's eggs from which the nucleus had been extracted. Then the stem cell would contribute the full complement of 46 chromosomes needed for a human life. Together with the egg, it would constitute a new embryo, which could be implanted into the mother's uterus free of the defective gene.

At this point in time, reproductive cloning is very unsafe. The team of Scottish scientists led by Ian Wilmut needed 277 attempts at cloning in order to produce Dolly, its one success, in 1997.[4] Success rates in cloning mammals have not improved much since then. Deaths in utero are very common, and unhealthy animals sometimes come to term. Considerations of safety are sufficient to judge that it would be unethical to attempt reproductive cloning in human beings at this time. For those who do not oppose the animal experiments that could improve the state of the art and eventually make human reproductive cloning safe enough to attempt, the project may seem well worthwhile—perhaps especially where cloning would enable creation of healthy children with a biological link to parents who carry serious genetic defects.

Another approach to modifying the genomes of babies-to-be is very safe and free of the controversy surrounding reproductive cloning: genetic modification of gametes. Because sperm are so much more plentiful than ova, and procured more easily, sperm modification is especially promising. One of several gene modification techniques could be employed to introduce desired genetic material into the sperm population of a man whose genes include a disease-causing mutation. Then his sperm could be examined to find some that took up the desired genetic material. These could be used in efforts to achieve IVF, and the resulting embryo could be implanted into the mother's uterus. If the mother also carries a disease-causing mutation, one or more of her eggs could be similarly modified but, as mentioned, procuring eggs is more difficult.

A limitation of the genome-altering techniques described so far is that they require IVF. This technology is very expensive—typically almost $10,000 per cycle (attempt)—which is not surprising considering all that IVF involves: drugs to stimulate super-ovulation (to produce multiple eggs), retrieval of eggs, fertilization, incubation of embryos, and finally transfer to the uterus. The process also tends to be highly taxing and uncomfortable for women. Two possible developments, though, could make IVF much more attractive, on balance, clearing the path for more widespread use of this method of achieving fertilization.

One possible development is an improved method of freezing eggs. Egg freezing is currently hindered by a distortion of structures inside ova that is caused by the expansion of water when ova are frozen. If this problem is overcome, many women might be interested in freezing a supply of viable eggs—and then thawing and using them for IVF after recovering from an illness, getting tenure, or finding partners with whom they want to raise children. (The creation and freezing of *embryos*, after fertilization, is also possible, but this option may be unattractive to women who would like to raise a child with a partner but have yet to find the right person.) Egg freezing not only allows women to control the timing of their pregnancy in the way described; it also stops the aging process that eventually makes eggs unviable. As of today, though, the only way to procure multiple eggs at one time is to undergo drug-stimulated superovulation.

A second possible development would expand options. In vitro *egg maturation*, as Ronald Green explains, would overcome current biological limits on the production of ripe eggs:

This technology, already being attempted with mouse eggs, mimics the process that already takes place each month inside the ovaries when, from the stock of hundreds of thousands of immature eggs, the body chooses one or two of them to ripen for fertilization. [W]ithout the expense or difficulties of drug stimulation, a young woman could undergo a onetime, outpatient biopsy and put aside a small slice of ovarian tissue containing hundreds or thousands of tiny, immature eggs for freezing. When she is ready to start her family, a few of these eggs could be thawed and matured in vitro to the point where they could be fertilized with her partner's sperm. If the procedure does not work, she would still have an ample supply of eggs on hand to try again.[5]

Egg freezing and in vitro egg maturation are likely to make IVF more attractive to many women.

These techniques of the future, together with sperm modification and/or various methods for changing an embryo's genome, could usher in an age in which many couples have an ample supply of sperm, eggs, and even embryos in a laboratory, where PGD can be used for selection purposes. There is nothing very far-fetched, scientifically, about this scenario. The genetic control it would confer on prospective parents would enable not only selection of embryos with desired traits and the more direct intervention of PGT. It would also make PGE a far more realistic possibility.

Before proceeding to our ethical exploration of PGD, PGT, and PGE, let us recall several conclusions from Chapter 2 that will be highly relevant to our discussion. Regarding our origins, we concluded with some uncertainty. It was argued that we are essentially human organisms and not essentially minds or persons, with the consequence that we come into being early in gestation, long before a fetus becomes sentient. I defended the view that we originate as early as the 16-cell stage, when differentiation of cellular function begins a few days after conception, and as late as when spontaneous twinning and fusion are precluded, around two weeks after conception. I also acknowledged that my arguments left room for doubt, and that the view that we originate at the time of conception is a reasonable contender. The issue of when we originate is worth flagging because the possibility of altering genes raises questions about whether the individual whose genes are altered and the individual who benefits later are one and the same individual.

Several of the ethical conclusions reached in Chapter 2 are especially relevant to this chapter. I argued that the moral status of embryos did not preclude their use in research that would entail their destruction. While acknowledging the reasonableness of a pro-life view that would condemn such research as immoral, I contended that the most ethically appropriate *policy* response to ontological and moral pluralism regarding prenatal human life included the legal permissibility of embryo research—and abortion at least until the time of fetal viability. Accordingly, this chapter will proceed on the assumption that embryo research should be legally permitted. This is important because the prospects for successful PGT and PGE depend heavily on embryo research. Moreover, use of pre-implantation genetic diagnosis for selection purposes may entail the destruction, or at best neglect, of embryos not selected for implantation; and use of the older testing methods of amniocentesis and CVS are often followed by abortion in the first two trimesters. With this normative background, the ethical analysis to follow will focus on issues other than those addressed in Chapter 2.

PRENATAL GENETIC DIAGNOSIS, SELECTION, AND DISABILITY

PGD includes the testing of fetuses with amniocentesis or CVS, of embryos prior to implantation, and of gametes. By far, the most significant and well-developed set of objections to PGD has been advanced by disability advocates. As noted earlier, PGD can be used either for the purpose of negative selection (selection against an undesired trait) or for positive selection (for a desired trait). So far, however, actual use of PGD has mostly served negative selection: Existing tests target genetic diseases (with the exceptions of gender and tissue compatibility). Moreover, issues raised about positive selection are primarily issues about PGE itself, the topic of a later section. And disability advocates' moral objections to PGD mostly focus on negative selection. So this discussion will do so as well.

Three objections are especially prominent: (1) the loss-of-support argument, (2) the expressivist objection, and (3) the thesis that so-called disabilities are really just differences. The third objection will motivate a careful consideration of how we should conceptualize disability. For now, we will proceed with an intuitive understanding of the term: A disability is a biologically based condition of an *individual* (not of her circumstances) that limits functioning in a significantly disadvantaging way. Familiar examples of disabilities that have a genetic basis are cystic fibrosis, Huntington's disease, Alzheimer's disease, and some forms of deafness, blindness, and mental retardation.

The Loss-of-Support Argument

According to this objection, widespread use of PGD to select against gametes, embryos, or fetuses with genetic predispositions to disability will reduce the number of persons with disabilities. This reduction in numbers, in turn, is likely to reduce the amount of financial, logistical, and social support available to persons with disabilities. For this reason, use of PGD for negative selection is, at best, a morally troubling practice that should be discouraged and, at worst, a morally indefensible practice that should be banned.

Of the three major disability-related objections to PGD, this is the least compelling. First, it is hardly inevitable that a reduction of numbers of persons with a particular disability will result in decreased support for them.[6] Such measures as public education about the disability in question, and a commitment to public funding for research on the disability and for logistical support for affected individuals, might not only prevent loss of support of relevant kinds; they might increase such support.

Second, if the reasoning of the loss-of-support argument were sound, it should lead us—quite absurdly—to object to the *therapeutic elimination* of particular disabilities through medical means, physical therapy, and the like. For example, a cure for schizophrenia, if widely available, would reduce the number of persons with schizophrenia, but it would surely be misguided to oppose the development of such a cure on loss-of-support grounds. The same idea applies to medical interventions and forms of therapy that enable individuals with paralyzed limbs to overcome their paralysis.

Finally, even if it were predictable that widespread use of PGD would reduce support for persons with disabilities, and even if this reasoning did not have absurd implications regarding medical interventions and therapies for individuals with disabilities, it would not follow that use of PGD is wrong.[7] Loss of support for persons with disabilities is, of course, morally undesirable. But so are lost opportunities to help those who would benefit by avoiding disabilities. It would be the height of special pleading to claim that the loss incurred by already existing persons with disabilities automatically counts more than anyone else's losses. Everyone's interests matter. So even if we set aside the first and second replies to the loss-of-support argument, its proponents would have to do much more to advance a strong case against PGD. For they would need to show why the importance of preventing lost support for persons with disabilities proves to be the overriding consideration in view of other values at stake.[8]

The Expressivist Objection

A large, high-quality literature has emerged about what has come to be called "the expressivist objection."[9] The objection is given voice in such statements as these: "Do not disparage the lives of existing and future disabled people by trying to screen for and prevent the birth of babies with their characteristics"[10]; and "The message at the heart of widespread selective abortion on the basis of prenatal diagnosis is the greatest insult: some of us are 'too flawed' in our very DNA to exist; we are unworthy of being born. . . ."[11] Yet the so-called expressivist objection is really a family of closely related objections, or arguments—some presented in the literature, some voiced in public discussion—with different emphases and somewhat different targets. Sometimes it is the individual or collective *use* of PGD for negative selection that is faulted; sometimes it is the *medical institutions* that routinely promote and provide this technology for negative selection that come under criticism. Furthermore, the messages attributed to the choices, practices, or institutions in question vary somewhat in content. So there is some risk in trying to articulate the expressivist objection in a single statement. Nevertheless, this is how I understand it in a nutshell:

> The use or routine promotion of PGD for purposes of selecting against gametes, embryos, or fetuses that test positive for a genetically-based disability express several negative messages to disabled persons and the society at large. The messages expressed are roughly the following: *Disabilities are the most important features of individuals who possess them; these individuals, in virtue of their disabilities, have lives that are not worth living and/or not worth the burden they impose on their families and society; and these individuals, in virtue of their disabilities, have less moral worth than individuals who lack disabilities.* In expressing these messages, such use or promotion of PGD wrongs persons with disabilities by stigmatizing them, devaluing their lives, and denying their full and equal moral status.

According to many disability advocates, the expression of these messages is wrong for several reasons. First, like any other person, a person with a disability has innumerable traits and should not be "reduced" to her disability. Second, persons with disabilities can enjoy a very high quality of life—at least if others cooperate by not discriminating against them and not creating obstacles by designing buildings, communication systems, and the like solely for the convenience of "abled" persons. Third, the parents and family members of a disabled person need not experience an overwhelming burden of care; indeed, they tend to enjoy a rewarding family life and to cherish the disabled individual as much as other family members. Fourth, persons with disabilities have exactly the same moral status as persons lacking disabilities: the full and equal moral status of persons.

In replying to this argument, let me begin by noting that I accept all four claims advanced in the preceding paragraph. Accepting these claims, however, does not imply acceptance of the objection. For the latter rests on two further assumptions: (1) that use or promotion of PGD for purposes of negative selection necessarily expresses what the objection claims it expresses, and (2) that to express these messages wrongs persons with disabilities. Some who advance the expressivist objection may also assume (3) that, because expressing these negative messages wrongs persons with disabilities, PGD should not be made available. But this third assumption makes the objection harder to defend and is not what all proponents of this objection have in mind. Some, for example, hold that the proper conclusion to draw from the objection is that prospective parents have strong (whether or not conclusive) moral reason not to avail themselves of PGD for negative selection even if it is legally available; and even if, at the end of the day, PGD should be made available, it should not be routinely and aggressively promoted by medical institutions as it currently is.[12] So let us address only assumptions (1) and (2), which in the absence of (3) allow for a more modest, defensible position.

According to assumption (2), to express these negative messages wrongs persons with disabilities. Now, I agree with disability advocates that the messages attributed by the expressivist objection are unenlightened and perhaps morally obnoxious. It does not follow, however, that to express these messages wrongs persons with disabilities. If one sincerely believes the content of these messages, does it wrong persons with disabilities to express them? (Does it wrong animals to express views that underestimate their moral status if one holds the mistaken view sincerely?) I'm not sure. In any case, I will grant assumption (2) for the sake of argument. The reasoning under consideration founders on assumption (1), the claim that use or promotion of PGD necessarily expresses these hurtful messages.

If use or institutional promotion of PGD communicates anything, it does so nonverbally. Verbal communication, by contrast, involves a public language: a highly complex, rule-governed system of signs whose conventions of meaning are broadly accepted by the linguistic community in question. Verbal communication can be a highly precise means of communicating. More importantly here, its rules permit definite verdicts—not always but much of the time— about correct and incorrect usage. If Mom asks Joey whether he ate the cookies, his saying "no" means that he did not. He cannot say "no" and then, when evidence emerges and Mom cross-examines him about lying, claim that by "no" he means what other people mean by "yes." Words have *public* meanings.

Nonverbal communication is sometimes very determinate and at other times ambiguous. If another driver cuts me off, and I give him the finger with an angry facial expression, my meaning is clear. I am in no position to claim later that I was just conveying "Top of the morning!" to the other motorist. Giving the finger with an angry countenance, in that context, is to use a sign—the raised middle finger—in a way that conveys its usual meaning ("F you"). It does not leave room for an unusual reading (e.g., one of irony or mock anger if the context warrants such a message and the finger-giver smiles or presents an exaggerated expression).

The use of PGD, whether individual or collective, is not part of an agreed-upon system of signs.[13] What people mean or express through particular choices regarding PGD and associated actions such as non-selection of embryos or abortion is therefore, it would seem, relatively ambiguous. One might reply, however, by appealing to the philosophical thesis that intentional actions always imply general value judgments.[14] For example, to slaughter a turkey for Thanksgiving dinner implies the ethical permissibility of killing turkeys and the judgment that turkeys have less moral status than persons (assuming, as most do, that persons are not to be killed and devoured on holidays). In the same way, the disability advocate might argue, use of PGD for purposes of negative selection implies and expresses the messages identified earlier.

There are two flaws in this reply. First, when one acts in a way that one believes is *unjustified*—say, cheating on taxes out of moral weakness—one does *not* imply that doing so is justified. This point challenges the claim that every intentional action implies a value judgment. Now, presumably, most people who use PGD believe that their doing so is justified, so my second point addresses their situation: The judgments one implies through the relevant actions (assuming one implies something) are too ambiguous to permit an authoritative attribution of the messages attributed by the expressivist objection. Suppose you use PGD and select against embryos with a disposition to develop Huntington's disease. I grant that your choice has some sort of normative meaning—or range of meanings—in the sense that it cannot be said to mean *just anything* (e.g., "Break dancing is good exercise"). Nevertheless, the normative meaning of the act is far too open to reasonable interpretation for the expressivist objection to succeed.

To support my claim, I will reiterate, in italics, each of the messages ascribed in the objection and then offer an alternative reading in bold. So consider: (1) *Disabilities are the most important features of individuals who possess them.* **(1a) Disabilities can be relevant features of individuals in some contexts, including reproductive ones.** (2) *These individuals, in virtue of their disabilities, have lives that are not worth living and/or not worth the burden they impose on their families and society.* **(2a) It is reasonable to expect (fallibly) that the lives of persons with certain substantial disabilities, other things being equal, will feature a lower quality of life—or at least special hardships—for those who live them and/or pose greater difficulty for families and society than the lives of persons lacking the disabilities.** Here is a second alternative reading: **(2b) It is acceptable to prefer not to have a child with a particular substantial disability and to make reproductive decisions accordingly.** (3) *These individuals, in virtue of their disabilities, have less moral worth than individuals who lack disabilities.* **(3a) Persons with disabilities have full moral status, but fetuses do not.**

I submit that the alternative interpretations of the messages expressed by use of PGD for negative selection are perfectly reasonable interpretations and, moreover, that the messages they ascribe are neither unenlightened nor morally obnoxious.[15] If that is correct, then the expressivist objection fails to cast significant moral doubt on the use of PGD. The strongest reply available to one advancing this objection, I think, is to question the legitimacy of the alternative readings offered in (2a) and (2b). One might argue that it is a prejudice-driven error to judge that disability can be expected to impose a lower quality of life, or even special hardships, on the person who has it or an additional burden on the individual's family or society. For this reason, the reply continues, families do *not* have the prerogative to select against disabilities, so stating their preference to do so hardly justifies such a choice. Because the last point rests on the claim that the judgment stated in (2a) is erroneous, this claim is pivotal. It receives its strongest defense from the third major objection to PGD, the thesis that, contrary to popular belief, disabilities are merely differences. So the expressivist objection as it applies to the *use* of PGD can succeed only if the thesis that disabilities are merely differences proves justified. We will find out in the next section.

It remains now to consider the expressivist objection as directed against the routine, aggressive promotion of PGD. I have argued that prospective parents may use PGD for negative selection with a wide variety of attitudes about disabilities and their significance. If I am right (and my argument will not be complete until we conclude the next section), then this suggests that use of PGD for negative selection cannot be said to express a unified, morally unenlightened message of the sort attributed by the expressivist objection. By contrast, *routine, aggressive promotion* of PGD seems less compatible with a variety of moral attitudes including appropriate ones. It may be plausible to argue that medical institutions that promote PGD in this way socially express at least some of the meanings attributed in the objection, thereby wronging persons with disabilities. I will not examine the expressivist objection in relation to routine, aggressive promotion of PGD more closely than this because I am inclined to accept both the argument and its conclusion about wronging persons with disabilities. What clinics offering PGD ought to do (assuming PGD should be offered at all) is to engage prospective parents in an even-handed, unpressured, lengthy discussion of possible advantages and disadvantages of PGD *and of the rich, rewarding lives that persons with disabilities and their families so often enjoy.* Somewhat analogously, though I will not defend the claim here, fertility clinics should engage prospective parents in an even-handed, unpressured, thorough discussion of possible advantages and disadvantages of various forms of assisted reproduction *and of the humanitarian and other advantages associated with adoption.*

Thus, I conclude this section by noting that the expressivist objection may well succeed against routine, aggressive promotion of PGD whereas it fails against the use of PGD—unless the thesis that disabilities are mere differences proves successful.

The Thesis That Disabilities Are Really Just Differences

According to a third prominent disability-based objection to PGD, so-called dis-abilities are really just differences in functioning from those considered normal.[16] Such "disabilities" as dyslexia, blindness, deafness, and paraplegia are not *inherently* disadvantageous any more than being non-Caucasian is inherently disadvantageous. Disadvantages are due to the context in which the relevant conditions exist, contexts that often prominently feature discrimination and a lack of consideration on the part of the "abled" majority. Any disadvantages, that is, are contingent; they are not a necessary consequence of an objectively bad condition.

Whether a given condition is perceived as a disability, the argument elaborates, depends on the context, environment, and existing social arrangements. Unless one wants to be a pilot, color-blindness generally goes unnoticed by others and is not considered a disability. But if traffic lights placed green and red lights in varying configurations so that colorblind people could not distinguish them, their ability to drive safely would be greatly impaired and they might be regarded as disabled. Dyslexia is considered a significant disability only where reading is expected. Before reading was part of human culture, the same physical condition was probably not noticed, much less considered a handicap. Deafness is considered a disability by a hearing majority that uses spoken language and telephones. But deafness is really just a difference—one that need not pose disadvantages in certain environments. If everyone signed rather than spoke and texted rather than called by telephone, the hearing majority might not consider deafness a disability. Indeed, if our world were filled with loud, varying noises that consistently distracted hearing persons, the ability to hear might count as a disability.

So disabilities, according to the argument, are just differences. PGD is used almost exclusively to identify these differences with the intention of not bringing into existence individuals who would feature them. Such selection against disabilities is a form of unjust discrimination, analogous to selecting against certain races. It reflects and reinforces a pernicious prejudice against persons with disabilities. Therefore, use of PGD should be disallowed or at least strongly discouraged.

This argument provokes three questions: (1) What is a disability? (2) Are disabilities inherently disadvantageous? (3) What do the answers suggest, ethically, about PGD? Let us take up these questions in turn.

WHAT IS A DISABILITY?

The argument based on the thesis that disabilities are just differences rejects one model of disability and asserts another. According to the *medical model*, a disability is a relatively long-lasting, biologically grounded condition of an

individual that impairs functioning in one or more significant ways. On this
mainstream conception of disability, it is the individual's condition itself that
causes significantly impaired functioning. Being blind, for example, is a disability because it precludes one from the undeniably important function of
seeing. The *social model* of disability, by stark contrast, maintains that disability involves a loss or limitation of opportunities to participate in valued
activities or forms of community life due to institutional or social barriers. In
other words, disability is socially constructed. Many have found the social
model to offer a helpful corrective to the naïve simplicity of the medical
model, yet also to exaggerate in claiming that disability is entirely a social
construction. Such thinkers favor a more moderate *interactive model* of disability: disability as a product of the interaction between biological dysfunctions of an individual's mind or body—often called *impairments*—and the
social and physical environment in which the individual exists.[17]

Proponents of the social model of disability and the thesis that disabilities are
just differences are surely correct that what we classify as a disability is not solely
a matter of biological dysfunction. Only certain inabilities will even interest us
as dysfunctions. For example, no human being can see ultraviolet light, so inability to do so does not count as a disability. If many humans could see ultraviolet light and this ability were crucial to reading the texts used in schools, the
inability would probably count as a disability. We considered other examples
earlier. I take it that they and similar examples demonstrate the inadequacy of
the medical model. But the social model has competition from the more moderate interactive model. If the latter is more accurate, then what counts as a
disability is partly a matter of an objective impairment: a biological dysfunction.

It may seem obvious that the interactive model is correct on this point. Who
could deny that blindness is a disability that involves impairment of one's visual
system? But even this seemingly obvious example of objective impairment may
not be so simple. A proponent of the social model might assert the following:

> We count blindness as a disability but ordinary near-sightedness as just an
> inconvenience. But that is because effective eyeglasses are readily avail-
> able, whereas we do not have a technology, much less one readily available,
> that compensates so thoroughly for blindness. With different funding and
> social priorities, we might have such a technology, in which case blindness
> would be seen as an inconvenience rather than a disability.

A proponent of the interactive model may respond by insisting that, regardless of society's choices, blindness is a physical characteristic of an individual
that prevents normal human functioning of a sort that is undeniably important
to creatures like us: vision. She might add that nearsightedness *is* a disability,

but in present circumstances (at least where eyeglasses are widely available) a trivial one. Similarly, even if a perfect cure for blindness were discovered and provided to all who needed it, blindness would remain a disability, albeit a trivial one. Inability to see is an objective impairment in humans, who normally see, even if it is not in bats, who do not. This response acknowledges that the present conception of disability uses *normal human functioning* as a reference point. It might even allow—indeed, it should allow—that widely shared *values* play a role insofar as an impairment of normal human functioning counts as a disability only if it is forecloses *valued* functionings. As Jonathan Glover puts it, it would not count as a disability if one's toenails lost the capacity to grow.[18]

A champion of the social model will now press the issue of values. Widely shared values, which serve as an essential reference point in identifying disabilities, are a social phenomenon—consistent with the view that disability is socially constructed. A proponent of the interactive model, however, may reply that the values relevant to the identification of disability are not as contingent, arbitrary, and malleable as the term "socially constructed" suggests. At least in the case of the most severe disabilities, the types of functioning they prevent or impair are—from a human perspective—undeniably important. These disabilities, the argument continues, *by their very nature* interfere with opportunities for human well-being. This assertion takes us to our next major question.

ARE DISABILITIES INHERENTLY DISADVANTAGEOUS?
AN EXCURSION INTO VALUE THEORY

If disabilities are inherently disadvantageous, they do not simply reflect different ways of functioning. The issue requires a brief excursion into *prudential value theory*—*value theory* for short—which features competing accounts concerning what, at the most basic level, constitutes individual well-being or flourishing. Such an account offers a view about what counts as a benefit, what counts as harm, and what makes an individual's life go better or worse from the standpoint of her own interests.

Value theories can be grouped, at a general level, into subjective accounts and more objective accounts. Subjective accounts understand our well-being to be ultimately a function of our having certain valuable mental states and avoiding contrary mental states. Classical hedonists, for example, argued that well-being is happiness, where the latter was equated with pleasure (in all its many varieties) and the absence of pain (in all its varieties).[19] Responding to the point that we generally value things in addition to pleasurable or agreeable mental states, an alternative subjective approach construed our well-being in terms of the satisfaction of our desires or preferences—the objects of which typically included not only agreeable feelings, but also states of the world such as achieving something or having friends.[20] Because we sometimes desire things that do not prove conducive to our welfare, some theorists refined this approach so that our well-being was a function of the satisfaction of those desires we would have *if adequately informed*. But this theory, too, proved problematic. For one thing, we might have an informed desire for something—such as being promoted—and then find, when this desire is satisfied (when we get what we wanted), that *we* are not. If the satisfaction of an informed desire does not give us any *felt* satisfaction, it is unclear why it should count as valuable on a subjective account. Moreover, an informed desire might be satisfied—what you want happens—without your being aware of it; indeed, you might be dead when it happens. Suppose, for example, you have a single conversation with someone while traveling, form the desire that he succeed in his quest to earn a degree, and never communicate with him again. If it turns out that he does earn a degree, then your desire has been satisfied and, according to the informed-desire theory, your well-being has ipso facto improved. But there is something odd about a theory that suggests that you benefit from such remotely satisfied desires. Your well-being seems more closely tied to what happens in *your* life and, arguably, only in ways that affect your *experience*. It is open to the informed-desire theorist to amend the theory such that only some restricted range of desires are relevant to the agent's well-being. Such amendments, however, raise a question: Is well-being really a function of satisfying desires per se? Or is it a function of quality of life, as hedonism suggests, or of factors that are more independent of the subject's mental life?

Taking up the latter possibility, some theorists defend more objective accounts of human well-being. I say "*more* objective" because it is widely appreciated today that any plausible account will have to have some subjective elements—allowing, for example, that enjoyment generally promotes well-being and allowing room for individual differences in temperament, taste, and nature in determining what makes a particular individual well-off. These accounts are significantly objective in maintaining that certain human activities, forms of functioning, or states of affairs are intrinsically valuable for one—irrespective of the pleasure, enjoyment, or satisfaction they bring a given individual, and whether or not he prefers them. For example, it is sometimes argued that one is better off, other things being equal, if one has deep personal relationships, accomplishes something, achieves understanding of important matters, lives autonomously, and experiences enjoyments.[21] A recent trend has been to characterize these and other allegedly objective components of human well-being in terms of *capabilities* to function in various ways.[22] In an effort to show that their approach is not implausibly remote from human experience, theorists of this stripe maintain that objectively valuable components of human well-being are such that people *characteristically* desire them and find them satisfying even if there are exceptions.

Subjective accounts of well-being clear more conceptual space than do objective accounts for the thesis that disabilities are mere differences. On subjective accounts, a given disability need not be disadvantageous for a particular individual even if it is disadvantageous for most people. Perhaps it is true that blind people experience more frustration and suffering, on average, than sighted people for reasons connected with their blindness. But if a given blind person is just as happy (however this concept is defined) as the average sighted person—and just as happy as he was before becoming blind (if the impairment was acquired)—there is no basis for judging his well-being to be lower just on account of blindness. If it does not make him less happy, it does not make him worse off, according to the subjective theorist. Moreover, the fact, if it is a fact, that blind—or deaf or paraplegic—people tend to be less happy than their "abled" counterparts has plenty to do with social arrangements, institutions, and attitudes that could be improved. So, even if some group of disabled people is less well-off *now*, that is likely to be a contingent fact rather than a necessary consequence of their disability.[23]

By contrast, an objective theorist—especially one who emphasizes functioning or capabilities—is more likely to judge major disabilities as per se injurious to well-being. To be unable to see is to be unable to function in an important way that is not only instrumentally valuable—helpful for many things we want or need to do—but also intrinsically valuable. To be unable to walk is not only enormously inconvenient; it also deprives one of an intrinsically valuable activity.[24]

It is an important fact that many persons with major disabilities deny being unhappy with them. Indeed, some insist that they are happy to be living a life characterized by their disability, that their experience with disability has added something valuable to their lives.[25] What should we make of these positive self-reports? According to the objective theorist, we must take into account the phenomena of *self-deception* and *adaptation*, which can distort a disabled (or otherwise disadvantaged) person's self-assessments of well-being. We deceive ourselves when we permit ourselves to believe something we would like to believe despite strong evidence against it. A disabled person may talk herself into the belief that she is faring just as well as she would without the disability, but this self-assessment is unreliable. In cases where individuals *lose* functioning as a result of illness or accident, adaptation is common: After an initial period of frustration and felt loss, the individual adapts to his new circumstances and, in time, reports increasing satisfaction with his life, sometimes to the point of feeling as well as he did prior to the loss of functioning. These cases may involve self-deception. Very commonly they involve a *lowering of expectations* such that one comes to have desires (e.g., to get outside in any way possible) that are easier to satisfy than earlier desires (e.g., to run vigorously).

Analogously, a very stoical prisoner may shed old desires for liberty and take solace in modest victories such as getting a decent sleep or not being harassed all week. But even if he feels as satisfied with his new lot as he was with his old, he is, according to the objective theorist, worse off for being confined.

Thus, one of the most significant challenges to subjective theories, and the view that disabilities are mere differences, is the assertion that certain activities such as seeing, hearing, and taking a walk are objectively, intrinsically valuable. In the face of optimistic reports from some persons with disabilities, this claim of objective value receives support from the stress on self-deception and adaptation. And the claim implies that disabilities that preclude such objectively valuable activities necessarily, to some extent, diminish well-being.

Against current trends in the value theory literature, however, I submit that the best possible subjective theory is more plausible than any objective theory. To motivate this claim, consider the rather bold assertions to which an objective theory is committed. Consider, first, its tendency to second-guess the positive self-assessments that are often advanced by disabled persons. Of course, there is such a thing as self-deception, which can distort one's optimistic reports, but we should attribute self-deception very cautiously. Generally speaking, it is the person herself who best knows how her life is going for her. Moreover, why should adaptation be considered an evaluative distortion? Yes, the satisfaction of modest desires tamped down by a loss of functioning—or any major setback—may be less of an achievement than the satisfaction of more ambitious desires, but this judgment of comparative achievement might not be relevant to the issue of *how well the subject's life is going for her*. Reassessing one's aims and making them more modest might be the wisest course in the face of loss or misfortune; and it is not obvious that one's new, lower baseline of expectation is necessarily a distorted baseline for determining well-being. I suggest that, if the blind person *really is* just as happy or satisfied as the sighted person, or if the prisoner *really is* as happy now as she was prior to imprisonment, there may be no reason to judge that in each case the former is less well-off than the latter, and that the absence of functioning in each case (sight, liberty) is injurious to the individual's well-being.

In addition to being presumptuous in second-guessing stoical individuals' self-reports, I suggest, the objective approach is theoretically presumptuous. Or, at any rate, it carries a heavy burden of justification. For objective theories assert the existence of standards of well-being that are to apply to individuals irrespective of whether those individuals care about the standards or resonate experientially with them. Why should those standards be authoritative in evaluating the well-being of individuals who do not embrace them? Individuals, after all, have a subjective sense of how their lives, or portions of their lives, are going, and well-being is a property of an individual, so there is a reasonable (rebuttable) presumption in favor of accepting individuals' self-assessments of well-being. Now consider, for example, an unambitious person who seems perfectly happy with his life, yet is judged by an objective theorist to be less well-off for lack of accomplishment—even though he does not desire accomplishment and correctly believes that it would not make him happier. It is no doubt true that most people find accomplishment satisfying. But, for one who does not, it is unclear that his life, lacking accomplishment, is less good *for him*. I do not claim that the objectivist's assertion is unintelligible or conceptually incoherent. Rather, I claim that it is a bit odd and stands in need of a strong justification—which, in my opinion, no one has ever supplied. By contrast, the fact that something such as accomplishment or friendship makes a given person happier and more satisfied certainly seems to be evidence that it makes her better off, consistent with subjective accounts.

One motivation for objective accounts is the perception that subjective accounts have insuperable difficulties. Here I will identify and reply to what I believe to be the three most significant challenges. Doing so will provide a preliminary sense of what the strongest possible subjective theory would look like. The first major challenge is to define happiness in some way that is more plausible than the usual reduction to either pleasurable feelings or desire-satisfaction. The second major challenge is to avoid a seemingly absurd implication of subjectivism: that a person who is happy only because all of her beliefs are systematically and profoundly distorted is well-off.[26] The third major challenge has already been touched upon but can be amplified. Not only disabilities and difficult circumstances but also social oppression and subordination can cause an individual to constrict her expectations and desires self-protectively. But doing so, according to the challenge, distorts such desires—even if they are adequately informed—as a benchmark for assessing well-being. A slave, accustomed to a life of profound subordination, may have very modest desires that are satisfied and may feel satisfied, but such satisfaction obscures the assault on well-being that slavery entails.

In response to these challenges, I offer three suggestions. The first is to define happiness not in terms of agreeable sensations or desire-satisfaction but as *life-satisfaction*: satisfaction with how one's life on the whole is going for one.[27] Much of the attraction of hedonism derives from the plausibility of the idea that an individual's well-being is determined by his happiness in some sense of that term. But reducing happiness to agreeable sensations is clearly too shallow to capture our understanding of human well-being. Meanwhile, desire-satisfaction, as we saw, is often too remote to do justice to our sense of what happiness or well-being involves, even if only informed desires count. We left open the possibility that only some range of informed desires should count—perhaps those whose satisfaction will affect our own lives and our experience—but that leads us to ask whether it is not desire-satisfaction (with certain qualifications) itself that constitutes our well-being but something more basic. To cut to the chase, I suggest that the reason the satisfaction of desires so often seems to contribute to our well-being is precisely because it contributes to our overall (subjective) sense that our lives our going well for us, a sense that in ordinary cases causes us to *feel* a kind of satisfaction. Happiness, in short, is life-satisfaction. Well-being is closely related to happiness, thus understood.

The second suggestion is to include a *reality-based* requirement for well-being. A person's happiness makes her well-off only if it is based on a more or less accurate understanding of her circumstances. With this requirement, a person whose happiness rests on thoroughgoing delusion is not well-off. The reality-based requirement makes the present subjective theory far more plausible by deflecting the unpalatable implication that one whose life is characterized by happiness-inducing delusions is well-off just because she is happy.[28]

The third suggestion is to accept the victory of stoicism. If a slave is happy despite having no illusions about his situation, then he has overcome the odds and is actually doing well. He is not less well-off just because his desires and expectations have been partly shaped by oppression. Oppression can tamp down a person's desires so that he aims for less than he otherwise would aim for and is satisfied with less than he would otherwise require in order to be satisfied. Our slave, let us say, would be delighted to be set free but, seeing little prospect for freedom, no longer suffers from an unfulfilled desire to be free. He feels relatively satisfied with more modest goods such as the friendship of other slaves, a clean dwelling to live in, a little bit of free time, and physical health. He completely understands his circumstances, including the injustice of being enslaved. Given his lack of self-deception, we should judge that he is doing well to the extent that he is satisfied with his life. While objective theorists would say that his lack of freedom makes him less well-off, regardless of how satisfied he is with his lot, the stoic (and perhaps the Buddhist) would disagree, applauding the way in which he has not allowed his happiness to be tethered to circumstances beyond his control. All I can say at this point in this brief discussion is that I find the stoic's judgment in a case like this to be more enlightened and believable. Accordingly, I suggest that the happy, undeluded slave is doing well despite being enslaved. (I am anxious to add, however, that *this judgment in no way justifies slavery*. The slave's rights have been violated no matter how well he is doing.)

With this theoretical discussion in hand, let us finally return to the questions of whether disabilities are inherently disadvantageous and what the answer suggests about PGD. If I have been right to endorse a subjective theory of well-being over any objective approach, then it follows that—in one important sense—disabilities need not be disadvantageous. A person can be disabled and fare just as well, overall, as a person who occupies identical circumstances except for lacking the disability; the disability per se is not inimical to her overall well-being. It does not follow, however, that disabilities are mere differences. I do not believe that they are.

Disabilities involve the absence of a kind of functioning that plays a significant role in human life. To be blind, for example, is to "begin" with a disadvantage. Being able to see is a massive advantage. Sighted people treasure the ability to represent the world visually and presumably find some (subjective) intrinsic value in visual experience. Now, someone who has *never had* vision may not lose out, in terms of intrinsically valued experiences, from not seeing—just as we do not lose out from not seeing ultraviolet light and not experiencing bat-like sonar.[29] But the *instrumental* value of vision to human beings across the board, in the world as we know it, is enormous, and this fact has an irreducibly biological (as opposed to social) basis: Animals evolved vision because it is so helpful for navigating. To be sure, through adaptation and self-discipline, a blind person may manage to be just as well off as a typical sighted person—but to do so is to beat the odds and overcome the instrumental disadvantage. So we might say that disabilities are (1) *presumptively* disadvantageous in the sense of presenting an obstacle (even when social accommodations are abundant), but (2) *not necessarily* disadvantageous in that some persons with disabilities, despite their obstacles, fare as well as their "abled" counterparts or, in the case of acquired disability, as well as they themselves fared prior to becoming impaired. Importantly, these persons with disabilities are not less well-off than their level of (informed) happiness suggests.

Because disabilities are *presumptively* disadvantageous, it must be considered harmful to inflict a disability on an individual.[30] Typically, even with appropriate social accommodation, disabilities reduce opportunities and create burdens for those who bear them, causing frustration and reducing satisfaction. This suggests what is valuable in objective accounts: They identify conditions, types of function, and states of affairs that—generally speaking in the world as we know it and with human beings as we know them—tend to make life go well. Objective theorists are right that having close personal relationships, accomplishing things, living autonomously, and certain forms of physical and mental functioning generally make a human life go better. Their error is to overgeneralize by claiming that these conditions and forms of functioning *necessarily* make a human life go better and that their absence *necessarily* makes a life go less well. If this is correct, then the value of objective accounts is that they provide *a presumptive list of welfare-conducing conditions*—which our social policies and parental decisions should generally support.

At the same time, we must not forget to listen carefully and openly to persons with disabilities when they talk about their quality of life and their interests. As disability advocates have convincingly argued, those of us who lack major disabilities tend to make the following errors: (1) underestimating the quality of life of persons with disabilities; (2) failing to appreciate the ways in which social and institutional choices can make their situation more difficult than it needs to be; and (3) perceiving persons with disabilities primarily in terms of their disabilities, rather than perceiving them as individuals with myriad characteristics of interest and importance. A major take-home lesson of any engagement with issues concerning disabilities is that, even if we have made some strides in recent years, we have quite a ways to go in the direction of overcoming these errors.

BACK TO PGD

Where does this leave us with respect to PGD? Although disability advocates who oppose PGD are correct that individuals born with disabilities often flourish, it remains true that (nontrivial) disabilities pose substantial obstacles and typically make life more challenging for the individual in question and others who care for her—even with reasonable supports and accommodations. Given our earlier conclusions about prenatal moral status and the appropriate legal permissibility of abortion, there is a very strong moral presumption in favor of permitting PGD for purposes of negative selection. The considerations supporting the partly enlightened, partly exaggerated thesis that disabilities are just differences do not make a compelling case for overturning this presumption.

PRENATAL GENETIC THERAPY, ROBUST IDENTITY, AND BENEFIT

PGD is a clinical reality. So is genetic therapy on already-born persons, though this mode of medical treatment is considered experimental in all its forms. Since commencement of the first genetic therapy trial in 1990, progress has been slow, but completion of the Human Genome Project accelerated advancement in the basic science underpinning the field.[31] In contrast to PGD and postnatal genetic therapy, *prenatal* genetic therapy is only a future prospect. It may not be very far off, however, as suggested by the earlier description of how reprogenetics might be expected to develop (see "Background" in this chapter).

We may distinguish three types of PGT. As discussed earlier, therapy could be performed on *gametes* prior to fertilization or on *embryos* prior to implantation. A third type of PGT would be performed on *fetuses* by injecting desired genetic material. Why wait until the fetal stage rather than intervening earlier? One possible motivation is a cautious desire to avoid therapeutic changes, while they are experimental, that are likely to be inherited by later generations; by inserting genetic material only into differentiated somatic cells, which will not be passed on to offspring, this goal would be served.[32] (Later I will question the rationality of this goal.)

Now, unless an attempted PGT would *benefit* a particular prenatal individual, it is not really therapy. Perhaps an attempt would fail to produce the desired effect or would do so while also producing undesired, harmful effects that overwhelm any desired change. But perhaps an attempt would achieve the desired genetic effect, without any undesired effects, yet fail to benefit anyone. How is that possible? It could happen if (1) the intervention results in the origination of a different individual than otherwise would have originated, or (2) the intervention eliminates one individual and creates another in its place. In neither case would there be a pre-existing human being who survives to benefit from therapy. Quite a few authors have puzzled over these possibilities, which raise the issue of prenatal identity. We will address this issue before turning to less esoteric issues concerning benefit and harm.

Prenatal Identity and the Robustness Thesis

Clarification of prenatal identity will help us address not only PGT, but also PGE. We need to ask how much change is compatible with a given human being's origination or continued existence. This raises the issue of *individual essentialism*. In Chapter 2, we considered the issue of our essence: What are we, most fundamentally? I argued that we are essentially human animals or organisms, but that answer and the question about *us* pertain to *kind essentialism*: the question of what *we human persons* essentially are. What about one of us in particular? I am not just any old human organism. I am *this* one. You are of the same basic kind as I, yet you are essentially different from me as an individual. You are essentially, well, you. The fact that a particular human organism is essentially *that individual* is crucial to understanding prenatal identity.

Earlier we noted that there are different stages at which prenatal genetic interventions may occur: prior to fertilization, during the embryonic stage, or later in fetal development. Wherever we draw the line indicating the time at which one of us originates—at conception, the time at which twinning is precluded, or sometime in between—there is an important ontological-conceptual difference between interventions before and those after that time. (The line may even have breadth if we come into existence gradually, but here we can ignore this complication.) We will explore this ontological-conceptual difference before considering its possible moral importance.

After asking whether a particular person, such as Queen Elizabeth, might have had different parents in "another possible world"—that is, in a counterfactual situation—Saul Kripke answers negatively with a rhetorical question: "How could a person originating from different parents, from a totally different sperm and egg, be *this very woman*?"[33] In his highly influential discussion, Kripke suggests that a given individual could not have come into being, in a counterfactual situation, from different parents—or even from different gametes—than those from which she did, in fact, derive. That seems entirely correct. I would never have existed if the very sperm and egg from which I derived had never united in fertilization. (Thus it is absurd when Lisbeth's mother in *The Girl Who Played with Fire* says to her daughter, "I should have picked a better [biological] father for you."[34]) But from this insight about our origins it does not follow that I originated as a zygote, the immediate product of conception. While its existence was *necessary* for my existence—in this, the actual world, or any other possible world—it might not have been *sufficient*. If I am right that we originate some days after conception, then it was not sufficient for my existence, the zygote being a sort of precursor to me; if I am wrong on this point, then assuming some version of the biological approach to our essence and identity is correct, we may originate as early as conception (see Chapter 2).

Wherever we draw a line marking our origins, why does it seem obvious that none of us could have derived from a different set of gametes than those from which he did in fact derive? A promising answer will suggest that pre-origination genetic interventions are likely to be numerical-identity-affecting (*identity-affecting*, for short).[35]

The answer I suggest is partly motivated by thought-experiments such as the following. Suppose the very same sperm and egg from which you derived had united in fertilization, but right before that moment a mutation in one of the gametes slightly changed its genome. The mutation, though, was inconsequential, making no difference to later phenotype. Intuitively, it seems that, despite the slight change of genome, *you* would have originated in this counterfactual scenario. This verdict seems plausible even if we imagine a few pre-origination mutations so long as they are insignificant, producing little or no change to the later phenotype. If this is correct, then your identity does not depend on deriving from a zygote with *precisely* the same genome; rather, it depends on deriving from the same gametes and *virtually* the same genome. Why must the genome be virtually the same? Consider another scenario: The very same gametes from which you in fact derived did unite in fertilization, eventually leading to the birth of a child; but prior to fertilization, the nuclear DNA of the egg was replaced with that from another woman's egg. Although the same ovum (same at least in terms of its membrane and cytoplasm) was fertilized by your father's sperm, the genome was radically different. The resulting child in this scenario has a very different genetic constitution from yours and so, it seems clear, is not you.

What does all this suggest about pre-origination genetic interventions? Some pre-origination genetic modifications will be identity-preserving, permitting the same human being to originate as would otherwise have originated. But the very purpose of genetic therapy (or enhancement) is to render a change in genotype that *makes a substantial difference* to the later phenotype: for example, lack of predisposition to a terrible disease. This suggests that any successful pre-origination genetic intervention will effect a genetic change that matters and will therefore be identity-affecting, resulting in the origination of a distinct human organism than otherwise would have originated.

Now consider genetic interventions that take place after one of us has already originated. How sensitive is post-origination identity? I submit that it is not very sensitive at all, that a post-origination human organism can survive many changes of genotype—including those likely to be pursued in real-world attempts at PGT and PGE. Call this the *Robustness Thesis*. What is its basis?

Each of us is essentially a particular living human organism. But, crucially, nothing in the idea of a particular living human organism seems incompatible with genetic—or, for that matter, environmental—modifications that change disposition to particular diseases, hair color, baldness, height, level of intelligence, athletic potential, or the like. Once one comes into existence, one can change greatly without going out of existence. As I child, I knew another boy who was badly injured in a car accident that caused him to be mildly mentally retarded. This event had a significant impact on his intellectual abilities and opportunities, and therefore on the life he led, but it did not kill him, or otherwise put him out of existence, and replace him with a disabled successor. Similarly, once you originate prenatally, you can change significantly—whether due to genetic modifications or factors in the uterine environment—without going out of existence. Once we exist, our numerical identity is robust and, in the world as we know, we do not go out of existence until we die (in the familiar sense of the term). So, when we change a lot, *we* change a lot. We change qualitatively, with possible implications for our narrative identity but not for our numerical identity.[36]

The Robustness Thesis implies that post-origination genetic interventions likely to be attempted in the name of therapy or enhancement will not be identity-affecting. Quite a few commentators, however, think otherwise. Why?

Some think PGT (or PGE) would be identity-affecting because they believe that we are essentially persons.[37] If we were essentially persons, then we would not originate until the human organism constituted or otherwise produced a person. On this view, any significant genetic modifications to the pre-personal organism would entail that a numerically different person came to be. Person essentialism was refuted in Chapter 2.

Others hold that prenatal identity is fragile for different reasons. One author claims that a stable genotype must be necessary for maintaining identity, with the implication that PGT "should be excluded from the notion of therapeutic intervention."[38] But his reasoning assumes that our identity, like that of a ship, is a matter of functional organization—which would be altered with significant genetic change.[39] It does seem plausible that an artifact such as a ship, built for a particular purpose, would have identity conditions that include its functional organization. If a ship is dismantled and its parts used to build a board walk, the ship no longer exists. But we are not ships or any other kind of purpose-given artifact. As a kind of living creature, I have argued, our identity over time is a matter of continuing one and the same life. This supports the Robustness Thesis.

Consider another possible basis for believing that prenatal identity is fragile, even after origination, as conveyed in this passage: "[T]he disease had a pro-found effect on the boy's identity. . . . [T]he immune deficiency caused by some genetic flaw severely limited activities, experiences, and interactions in which he could . . . participate. [So it was] surely an important factor in making him who he was."[40] One finds reasoning like this fairly often in the literature. It suggests that PGT could put its intended recipient out of existence by rendering a genetic change that would change who the resulting individual would be. But this inference seems to rest on a conflation, discussed in Chapter 3, of numer-ical identity and narrative identity. Certainly whether I have some terrible med-ical condition will affect who I am insofar as it affects my sense of self or narrative identity. But that does not entail the thesis that a genetic modification that prevents such a condition affects numerical identity. It does not, on my view, because once a human organism has originated, its identity is robust.

The Ethics of Prenatal Genetic Therapy

Commentators who believe that PGT is identity-affecting maintain that it does not benefit the individual on which it is performed: By affecting identity, PGD eliminates that individual and creates someone else in its spatiotemporal wake. If so, then the traditional purpose of medical interventions, benefitting the re-cipient of therapy, does not apply. Indeed, as there is apparently no individual who actually receives therapy (and survives) in PGT, it proves to be much less important than most medical interventions—and arguably a very weak candi-date for public funding. Moreover, for those who regard the recipient of PGT as having substantial moral status, there is a powerful reason *not* to perform PGT: It eliminates someone with substantial moral status.

In my view, as explained earlier, whether PGT is identity-affecting depends on the developmental stage at which it occurs. Prior to our origination, PGT is very likely to be identity-affecting, whether performed on gametes or (if we originate after conception) on the zygote-embryo. While one might infer that pre-origination PGT is for this reason morally wrong, or at least morally sus-pect, this inference would be premature. For, at this stage, PGT does not elimi-nate a being of our kind, a human organism that can develop into a human person. Instead, it prevents such a being from coming to be—just as contraception does. Since there is no serious moral objection to preventing a human individual from coming into existence, as opposed to eliminating an existing one, the fact that pre-origination therapy affects identity is morally insignificant. Such therapy harmlessly determines that a different human individual will originate than would otherwise have originated, rather than harming or otherwise affecting an existing human individual.

Moreover, there is a powerful moral reason in favor of pre-origination genetic therapy: If successful, it will prevent whoever does come into being from suffering from the targeted genetic disease or impairment. Because the therapy is identity-affecting, this benefit is not directed towards an already-existing individual. (Indeed, our use of the terms *therapy* and *benefit*, which normally imply a pre-existing individual whose condition is improved, is a little loose in this context.) Still, the therapy prevents significant suffering without harming anyone or violating anyone's rights. Assuming concerns about safety are responsibly taken into account, it would appear that pre-origination genetic therapy is morally acceptable, praiseworthy, and maybe sometimes even mandatory. If and when it is sufficiently promising from a technical standpoint, it will have a strong claim on public funding.

As the Robustness Thesis implies, once a human organism has originated, PGT is not identity-affecting. One and the same life will continue as the individual's genome is modified for therapeutic purposes. So the concern that (even post-origination) PGT constitutes a metaphysically odd form of eugenics—replacing a "defective" individual with a "better" one through genetic means—proves completely unfounded. Post-origination PGT, if it works, benefits its recipient. Other factors such as safety and technical feasibility being equal, it deserves the same social approval and support that other medical therapies enjoy.

Thus it turns out that while the point of our origination makes a large ontological-conceptual difference—identity is fragile before that point, robust after it—it makes no difference to the ethics of PGT. For different reasons, there is a strong moral case for PGT both pre- and post-origination. This is a convenient result because ambiguity about when we originate would otherwise make the ethics of PGT very confusing and uncertain.

One central ethical issue about PGT remains, however. It is often thought that, if any type of prenatal genetic modification is justified, it is *somatic-cell* PGT. The thought is that PGT is more justified than PGE and that somatic-cell interventions, which introduce genetic changes that are not inheritable, are more justified than germline interventions (on gametes, their stem-cell precursors, or undifferentiated embryos), whose effects are heritable. The essential concern about germline interventions is that they would magnify the risks involved in attempted genetic therapy. If the attempted therapy produces a harmful genetic error, it will be confined to one individual in the case of somatic-cell therapy, but it will be indefinitely inheritable in the case of germ-line therapy.[41]

Although very prevalent, this argument against germline therapy is fundamentally wrongheaded. While germline therapy would magnify any risks associated with a given procedure, it would also—in an exactly parallel way—magnify the benefits. If the benefit-risk ratio is favorable enough to justify an attempt at PGT, then it should be favorable enough to try it for a given individual and his or her prospective progeny. It is important to bear in mind a point that is routinely overlooked in discussions of PGT: While there are risks to attempting it, there are also risks to doing nothing.[42] To do nothing is to allow a disease or impairment to have its effects. It may be helpful to consider an example, provided by Ronald Green, of a potentially attractive germline genetic intervention:

> Since cells in the body die and are replaced by new, unmodified cells, even a somatic cell HIV/AIDS vaccine might require repeated administration. Imagine instead that we could invent a gene therapy suppository that a woman could use before intercourse, with or without her partner's consent. This would infect her sexual partner's sperm with a harmless virus carrying sequences to disable the [gene that causes susceptibility to HIV infection]. As a result, any child the woman conceives would have that change in all the cells of its body, including the sex cells. The result would be a generation of children who were naturally more resistant to HIV infection and would likely pass that resistance on to their children.[43]

This is an appealing prospect. (Technically, it involves enhancement because the intervention improves one's normal immune capacity, but it is hardly plausible that germline *therapy* would be less justified than germline enhancement.) Imagine, as well, a form of PGT that was designed to eliminate one's predisposition to develop Alzheimer's disease. If it is promising enough to try, I suggest, it is promising enough to try on the germline.

Germline PGT is, in general, no less justified than somatic-cell PGT. What justifies the latter justifies the former: a sufficiently favorable benefit-risk ratio, which by hypothesis is superior to the benefit-risk ratio of not deploying PGT. On the other hand, it may often be the case that, among the options with a sufficiently favorable benefit-risk ratio, the optimal strategy would be to proceed in stages as follows: Begin with somatic-cell PGT to see how the initial recipients fare and then, if they fare well, proceed to germ-line PGT. This strategy is especially likely to be preferable when the benefit-risk ratio, given current uncertainty, is only a little better than that of doing nothing. However, this cautious strategy might be indefensible in some cases, say, where the probability of successful therapy is very high and the disease to be avoided is especially devastating. In any case, the conventional wisdom that either condemns all germline genetic interventions or claims that they are less justified than somatic-cell genetic interventions across the board, is unsustainable.

PRENATAL GENETIC ENHANCEMENT

Is the PGT/PGE distinction morally important? Having discussed PGT, it remains to explore the ethics of PGE. In Chapter 3, we addressed the ethics of genetic enhancement but mostly limited the discussion to possible use by adults. The futuristic thought-experiments involving post-humans and post-persons, although implicitly involving PGE, focused not on the ethics of individual use of this procedure but rather on broader consequences of genetic enhancement pursued successfully over multiple generations. Our job now is to investigate the ethics of PGE per se. In doing so, we will not take up ethical issues—applying to genetic enhancement across the board—that were addressed in Chapter 3: issues pertaining to human identity, authenticity, human nature, human rights, or the security of humanity itself. Here we will consider doubts that PGE can be in the best interests of a child-to-be, concerns about parental attitudes that PGE may express, and residual concerns about effects on society.

Can PGE Be in a Child's Best Interests?

Obviously, with PGE it is impossible to obtain consent from the child-to-be. In pediatric medicine, because the young patient is considered incompetent to make informed, voluntary decisions for herself (and was not competent at any earlier time), the *best interests* standard is thought to be the appropriate decision-making guide. This reasoning extends beyond treatment to cases of enhancement.

Some doubt that PGE could *ever* be in the best interests of the child-to-be. Importantly, as suggested by our earlier analysis of identity-related concerns in connection with PGT, there are no *identity-based* grounds for the thesis that PGE is inimical to a child's best interests. If PGE is employed prior to the individual's origination, its modification of genetic information is likely to be identity-affecting, determining which possible individual will come into being. But because there is not yet a being of our kind—or of substantial moral status—in existence, it does not put such a being out of existence. Moreover, if successful, it has the advantage of ensuring that whoever comes into existence will have some desirable trait. If, on the other hand, PGE is employed after one of us has originated, it will (if successful) confer a benefit on that individual without affecting identity. In neither case is there an identity-based reason to doubt PGE's compatibility with a child's best interests. There are, however, two significant grounds for doubt: (1) the claim that genetic selection of a child's traits for nontherapeutic reasons violates her right to an open future, and (2) the belief that PGE would be unsafe.

THE RIGHT TO AN OPEN FUTURE

Some proponents of PGE maintain that *coming into existence* is itself a benefit and appeal to this thesis in developing their arguments.[44] But, in post-origination cases, PGE is performed on individuals who already exist, so in these cases PGE cannot possibly confer this alleged benefit. Moreover, the thesis that coming into existence is a benefit is notoriously controversial. We will return to it in Chapter 5. For now, I will assume nothing about the alleged benefit of coming into existence in replying to the two main grounds for thinking PGE to be incompatible with a child's best interests.

The first argument appeals to a child's right to an open future. In a highly influential discussion, Joel Feinberg argued that children have such a right.[45] The basic idea is that parents have an obligation to help their children develop capacities for autonomous choice and cultivate skills needed to afford them a wide array of options as to how to lead their lives as adults. Parenting that is overly constraining of children's options is said to violate their right to an open future (presumably, contrary to their best interests). How open must this future be? While Feinberg sometimes suggests that it must be *maximally* open, a more charitable interpretation of the basic idea is that the child's future should be kept *reasonably* open—that she should be afforded a reasonably wide array of options for how to live as an adult.[46]

The present concern is that PGE violates the future child's right to an open future by imposing the parents' will on the child regarding what traits she will have. It is one thing, the reasoning goes, to try to protect the child-to-be from disease or impairment with PGD; it is quite another to enhance intelligence, athletic ability, musicality, or the like. Typically, such enhancements reflect an overbearing parental desire for the child to lead a certain kind of life—such as intellectual, athletic, or musical. But parents owe it to their children to let them find their own way in life, not to lay down a definite path.[47]

This criticism of PGE assumes that children have a right to an open future. Do they? Consider parents who send their children to a Jewish or Catholic private school. Consider parents who require their children, from a young age, to train intensively in piano or tennis, a commitment involving hours of daily practice and the sacrifice of at least some enjoyments commonly available in childhood. These children are much more likely, when older, to participate in the religion of their upbringing rather than another (or no) religion, or to pursue a career in their chosen sport rather than a different sort of career. Have such parents violated their children's rights by so constricting their options?

In my view, that depends on details. If children who are sent to private religious schools are not brainwashed with dogma, and are afforded gradually increasing autonomy in their adolescence—with the possibility of changing their educational path if doing so seems more consonant with who they are—then their futures are, I think, left reasonably open. I would say the same about parents who arrange for intensive training in a sport or musical instrument so long as they do not allow this training to cause mental health problems or prevent the children from having some leisure, and so long as they are permitted to opt out at some point later in childhood. Parents who are involved in their children's lives have to make some choices about residence, schools, activities, lifestyle, and the like, and these choices will point their children in some directions rather than others. This, so far, is faultless. Indeed, it makes possible certain riches in their children's lives that would otherwise be unavailable. The point, again, is to permit a reasonably wide—not necessarily a maximally wide—array of options as an adult. A child whose parents prevented him from going to (any) school would violate his right to an open future. So would a parent whose religious indoctrination was so severe and dogmatic that the child predictably entered adulthood without the intellectual and psychological capacity to question the religion. And so would parents who ushered their children into a life of crime; doing so would likely create a future that was literally closed (behind bars).

PGE does not violate a future child's right to an open future by aiming to give him a particular trait. Using PGE to enhance for intelligence or athleticism does nothing to restrict a child's options. Of course, parents *could* choose PGE in the context of an overbearing parental plan and leave the children little choice except to become an academic, say, or an athlete. But this would be a case of bad parenting, which requires no PGE to exert its unfortunate effects.

So far I have argued that a child's right to an open future is compatible with PGE and some strongly directive parenting. "But," one might reply, "surely such parental control over a child's traits, being more heavy-handed than necessary for a child to grow up and have a good life, violates the child's best interests. It would be better for the child to have a maximally open future. Parents, as much as is humanly possible, should avoid imposing their dreams and agendas on their children." Actually, I doubt that a maximally open future would be best for a child; better, for example, to be morally influenced in such a way that one is unlikely to become an ax murderer or white-collar criminal. But there is a good point in the objection in that a future left only reasonably open might fall short of what is best for a child. I confess to being uncomfortable with levels of religious indoctrination that are commonly accepted in our society, and with the sort of parental driving that is often involved in the upbringing of children who become great musicians and athletes. But here, I think, we must distinguish between ideal parenting and acceptable parenting. To maximize a child's (good) options for the future is ideal, whereas to leave his future reasonably open is good enough.

How can that be right? Do parents not have an obligation to serve the child's *best* interests? Actually, I think not—if we are being literal and honest. The expression "best interests," whether used in the context of biomedicine or parenting, has always involved some hyperbole. The relevant standard, I suggest, is better described as protecting the child's *essential* or *vital* interests. To do so is the stuff of obligation, not merely an ideal. I deny that serving a child's (literally) best interests is strictly obligatory because there are too many mundane situations in which a parent can, acceptably, act a bit contrary to best interests. For example, the parents want to go out to dinner, the child would prefer not to, but the parents insist—and drive to the restaurant in the rain, imposing a very slight risk of a car accident, not to mention a gloomy meal, on their child. This may not be ideal from the standpoint of parenting, but it is certainly acceptable. It is compatible with protecting the child's essential interests. So is PGE, even if it comes with *some* expectations about the child's future, favoring some directions over others.[48]

If, as I suggest, we retain the entrenched phrase "best interests" and interpret it a bit loosely to mean "essential interests," then the preceding constitutes a persuasive rebuttal to the charge that PGE is incompatible with children's best interests because it violates their right to an open future. There remains the claim that PGE is inconsistent with children's best interests because it is excessively risky to the child-to-be.

CONCERNS ABOUT SAFETY

Thinkers who oppose genetic enhancements on grounds of safety often emphasize the absence of a precise vector for introducing genetic material into patients' bodies. The use of imprecise vectors, which deposits desired genes while leaving deleterious ones in place, creates much uncertainty about what will happen in a patient's body. This makes possible unanticipated genetic effects with unknown risks.

Concerns about risks are amplified in the prenatal context because we know far less about the technology of prenatal genetic interventions than the modest understanding we have about postnatal genetic interventions. Moreover, in the prenatal context the risk-benefit ratio of attempted genetic enhancements is likely, on average (not always), to be less favorable than the risk-benefit ratios associated with genetic therapy. Generally speaking, therapy responds to a highly problematic status quo, some impairment or disease or disposition thereto, so the benefits of successful therapy are quite considerable, very possibly outweighing the risks, especially if non-genetic options for treatment are lacking. But enhancement typically responds to a much more tolerable status quo—suboptimal functioning within a normal range—so the benefits of successful enhancement will tend to be smaller than those of therapy, with no expectation of proportionately reduced risk. (There are also what we might call "social risks" unique to enhancement, but we addressed some of these in Chapter 3 and will address others later in this chapter.) And, again, there is no possibility of obtaining consent from the individual to be affected by PGE—in stark contrast to the situation of competent adults making self-regarding decisions. While this is also true with PGT, the latter will often be in the affected individual's best interests where non-genetic treatments are unavailable. Thus, PGE is considerably more problematic than genetic enhancement for competent adults and at least some instances of PGT.

Nevertheless, there is reason to expect that that some forms of PGE will eventually satisfy the best-interests standard. Note, first, that the critics' emphasis on crude vectors for delivering genetic materials concerns the status quo of "gene addition"—the adding of genetic material to what is already present. Geneticists are working toward the development of more precise methods of gene correction and gene repair (see the earlier discussion of homologous recombination in "Background").[49] Another possibility under discussion is the construction of an artificial chromosome. Only with a much greater understanding of the realistic possibilities can we assess the possible benefits of genetic enhancement, an assessment that is needed for responsible risk-benefit assessments. Since the issue is empirical, there is a compelling case for permitting cautious research on techniques that might lead to genetic enhancements.

For now, let us use our imagination. Imagine that a type of PGT, whose target is a specific cognitive deficiency, has proven to be effective and safe. Meanwhile, a related form of genetic *enhancement*—augmenting an aspect of cognitive functioning in individuals deemed to be within the normal range—has proved effective and safe in competent adults. Next, an intervention that is ambiguous between therapy and enhancement (but promoted as therapy) proves effective and safe and then becomes widely used among teenagers and even children. But this is, let us suppose, the same intervention as what was classified as enhancement, though it is now used in a different population: those who show cognitive deficits but quite arguably fall within the normal range. Let us further assume that the benefits within this group and among those who lie clearly within the normal range are quite extensive, far exceeding the benefits of some previously (and appropriately) accepted genetic therapies. Next scientists propose to study what is essentially the same intervention, though now it would be administered prenatally, to fetuses lacking any known predispositions to cognitive deficits. This would be a case of PGE. It would be very similar to the postnatal enhancement and the PGT that already proved effective and safe. There are, as far as I can see, no compelling grounds for denying that such an intervention would be compatible with the affected individual's best interests. Let us therefore turn our attention to other leading objections to PGE.

Sufficient Regard for "Giftedness"?

One objection is articulated by Michael Sandel: "The problem with eugenics and genetic engineering is that they represent the one-sided triumph of willfulness over giftedness, of dominion over reverence, of molding over beholding."[50] Genetic enhancements, on this view, threaten our sense that children are gifts, not products to be designed. Openness to the unbidden, or unexpected, is essential to appropriate parenting, which requires acceptance of children for who they are.

The concern can be understood in terms of virtue ethics. Genetically enhancing our children-to-be, one might argue, would express a variety of bad attitudes and vices. These include arrogance (the opposite of humility), hyper-controllingness (as opposed to acceptance of the fortunes of life), avarice (rather than contentment with what is enough), and hyper-competitiveness in the case of parents who want their children to be better than other children. Parents ought to manifest virtues, not vices, in how they go about parenting. Accordingly, they should not opt for PGE even if their society makes it legally available.

This argument fails to show that there is anything inherently wrong with PGE. First, it begs the question to say that genetic enhancement is necessarily arrogant. In the absence of good reason to believe that it is God's job alone to perform genetic engineering, if we human beings are capable of doing so, it is unclear why it would be arrogant of us to make the attempt. As for the other vices mentioned earlier, they may or may not be involved in particular parents' interest in genetically enhancing their offspring. They need not be involved where parents simply want what is good for their kids. They can want this—and make sure their children have good educations and supportive environments— without being overly controlling about the direction of their children's development, without being greedy, and without caring much about how their children compare with other children.

Some parents, no doubt, will manifest some or all of these vices. But then the problem is the moral character of these parents. It is a problem that society has always had. I hope that we find ways to ameliorate it far better than we have so far—believing, as I do, that poor parenting abounds—but I do not see PGE as uniquely implicated in this problem. The desire to choose genetic enhancement for one's children-to-be need not reflect any bad attitudes at all.

Concerns about Positional Goods

Positional goods are goods whose value to an individual depends on comparisons with others. Scoring well on the Scholastic Aptitude Test, for example, is good for the test-taker insofar as many other students, with whom she is competing for acceptance into desirable schools, score less well. If her competitors all received the same score as she did, she would not benefit from her score. Consider another example. In swimming the freestyle, the ability to take multiple strokes without turning one's head to breathe—thereby saving time—while remaining adequately oxygenated is valuable to the extent that others lack this ability. If one took a drug that increased oxygenation efficiency, it would help one's performance in relation to competitors only if they did not procure the same benefit.

Positional goods may be contrasted with *intrinsic* goods, whose benefit to an individual is independent of comparisons with others. For example, if the pleasure I derive from listening to music is enhanced by meditating beforehand, meditation affords me a greater intrinsically valuable experience without disadvantaging anyone else. If a genetic enhancement allows me to focus on music in such a way that enhances my listening enjoyment, it too provides, or augments, an intrinsic good without disadvantaging others.

This same enhancement, however, may also confer positional goods if I am a musician who competes with other musicians for jobs and status, and the enhancement permits me to play better. Indeed, it is hard to think of an enhancement that could confer intrinsic goods without at the same time making possible certain positional goods. One might think that an enhancement that gave someone a sunnier disposition, making his life more enjoyable, would provide a major intrinsic benefit without conferring any positional goods. One might think again. For a sunnier disposition offers competitive advantages to politicians, salespersons, real estate agents, and others whose job performance is improved by extroversion and the expression of optimism. These reflections suggest that the distinction most relevant to our discussion is between enhancements that *primarily* confer positional goods and enhancements that *primarily* confer intrinsic goods. An enhancement that caused a sunnier disposition would fall into the latter group.

Positional goods create special problems in the context of enhancement. Consider the drug that enhances oxygenation efficiency, thereby allowing faster swimming. If even one person is known to use the drug, competitors have a reason to do so as well. But taking the drug may be unsafe, unpleasant, or expensive, not to mention against the rules. Those who decide to take it anyway may be responding to a degree of coercion—or at least heavy pressure to do what one would otherwise not want to do. Those who do not take the drug are treated unfairly by those who do. Although competitors have the option to identify cheaters to officials, this remedy is unavailable where it is unknown who is taking the drug. A possible solution, of course, is effective drug testing.

But what if a particular enhancement does not violate the rules? Such is the case with SAT prep courses. So many high school students applying to competitive universities take these expensive courses that equally ambitious students assume a risk by not taking a prep course. A kind of coercion is at work here for those who reluctantly register. For those who cannot afford it, there is a problem of economic fairness. Moreover, if everyone took the course, the result would be thoroughly self-defeating: Everyone would invest time, energy, and money without procuring any competitive advantage. In the status quo, as I understand it, the situation with respect to the SAT prep course is largely self-defeating among middle- and upper-class children, who can and do take the course, and unfair to lower-income children, who cannot afford it.

It is easy to see how genetic enhancements could create the moral problems associated with positional goods. Imagine parents who choose a form of PGE that confers the same advantage in oxygenation efficiency as the imaginary drug does. The parents, let us say, do not want to impose a swimming, running, or rowing career on their child—they are not so controlling—but want to confer this advantage in case the child is interested in such sports. Or, since relatively few people make their careers as competitive athletes, imagine parents who choose a form of PGE that confers a significant cognitive advantage that could be useful throughout school and in a broad range of careers. This sort of positional advantage would generate major concerns about coercion, fairness, and possibly collective self-defeat.

To some extent, we have this problem today with such positional goods as those conferred by excellent private school educations, expensive tutoring, specialty summer camps, and the like. These connect with problems of distributive justice: Against a background of distributive *injustice*—excessive, unjustified differences in resources between society's haves and have-nots—genetic enhancement available only to those who can afford them would exacerbate the injustice. The best solution is to *achieve* distributive justice with universal access to adequate health care, universal access to adequate schooling, and other appropriate social supports. With broad justice in the background, a prerogative to purchase additional advantages in schooling, medical treatment, or enhancements would probably be tolerable from the standpoint of justice—so long as the differences in advantages between the haves and have-nots are not permitted to grow excessively large.

This solution does not instruct us on how to proceed against the background of distributive injustice. Given that background, there is a case for not allowing further injustice through the purchase of PGEs that primarily confer positional goods. This case is strengthened in view of concerns about coercion: Parents will feel undue pressure to choose PGE for their children-to-be just to keep up with the genetic Joneses. The case for prohibition is weakened, however, by consideration of procreative freedom (a topic explored in greater depth in Chapters 5 and 6) and the discretion we usually afford parents to try to provide the best for their children. This prerogative is currently exercised when parents send their kids to elite private schools—when many children come from families unable to afford such an advantage, yet do not receive adequate schooling through the public system.

In view of all these considerations, there is a strong case for withholding public funding for PGE research or the clinical provision of PGE except in nations that have achieved universal access to adequate health care. The problem of positional advantage, however, is likely to arise in the form of individual purchases by wealthy families if and when PGE is perceived as safe and effective (possibly on the basis of privately funded research). Perhaps it would be justifiable to prohibit the purchase of PGEs that primarily confer positional advantages until major strides have been made in achieving justice in health care allocation, education, and the distribution of income and wealth. In the meantime, this approach would permit the discretionary purchase of PGE that primarily conferred intrinsic goods on its recipients.

A Final Concern: Promoting Stereotypes

Imagine a type of PGE that gave one's offspring lighter skin or straighter, thinner hair. We have reason to be very uncomfortable with the prospect of parents of color who would like their children to look "whiter" than they, the parents, do. Or imagine parents who wanted their daughter-to-be to have especially large breasts. In either of these scenarios, to opt for PGE is to embrace and reinforce discriminatory standards of beauty. Racism and sexism are such threats to social equality that I would recommend a prohibition of forms of PGE conferring changes such as those just described.[51]

Conclusion

The results of our investigation of the ethics of PGE may be quickly summarized. It was argued, first, that the best-interests standard provides appropriate guidance for parental decisions about PGE (and PGT) if interpreted as requiring protection of a child's *essential* interests. With that understanding, it was argued that some uses of PGE could both respect a child's right to an open future and be sufficiently safe to satisfy the best-interests standard. Next, the claim that PGE posed an excessive threat to our sense of children's "giftedness" was examined and found unpersuasive. The concern about positional goods, however, proved serious. It was argued that, so long as there is pervasive background injustice in the distribution of health care, education, and wealth, there should be no public funding for PGE research or the clinical provision of PGE. With some hesitation, I also suggested that a private market for types of PGE that would primarily confer positional goods should be prohibited until major strides have been made in overcoming distributive injustice. Finally, I recommended that society should prohibit forms of PGE that straightforwardly respond to, and thereby reinforce, blatant forms of racism, sexism, and other comparably invidious forms of discrimination.

NOTES

1. The presentation of factual background in this section has benefitted from President's Council on Bioethics, *Reproduction and Responsibility* (Washington, DC: PCB, 2004), chaps. 3 and 4, and especially from Ronald Green, *Babies by Design* (New Haven, CT: Yale University Press, 2007), pp. 42–52.
2. See GeneTests at http://www.geneclinics.org (accessed 6/22/11).
3. It is worth emphasizing here that I am following Green's lead (see note 1) in focusing on homologous recombination. More standard discussions, such as that of the President's Council on Bioethics (see ibid), tend to emphasize gene transfer: the insertion of genetic material in cells to replace or repair defective genes, add new genetic information, or regulate expression of genes. The major, well-known problem associated with gene transfer is the need to use an imprecise vector for introducing genetic material, as explained in chap. 3.
4. Harold Shapiro, "Ethical and Policy Issues in Human Cloning," *Science* 277 (July 11, 1997): 195–96.
5. *Babies by Design*, pp. 51–52.
6. Allen Buchanan, Dan Brock, Norman Daniels, and Daniel Wikler, *From Chance to Choice* (Cambridge: Cambridge University Press, 2000), pp. 266–67.
7. Ibid, p. 267.
8. A proponent of this objection might claim, in keeping with an argument addressed later, that disabilities are *not* inherently disadvantageous, in which case having an avoidable disability does not constitute a loss. I consider this claim later.
9. See, e.g., Buchanan et al., *From Chance to Choice*, pp. 272–81; James Nelson, "Prenatal Diagnosis, Personal Identity, and Disability," *Kennedy Institute of Ethics Journal* 10 (2000): 213–28; Erik Parens and Adrienne Asch (eds.), *Prenatal Testing and Disability Rights* (Washington, DC: Georgetown

University Press, 2000), Part III; Adrienne Asch, "Disability Equality and Prenatal Testing: Contradictory or Compatible?" *Florida State University Law Review* 30 (2003): 315–42, esp. 332–37; Jeff McMahan, "Preventing the Existence of People with Disabilities," in David Wasserman, Jerome Bickenbach, and Robert Wachbroit (eds.), *Quality of Life and Human Difference* (Cambridge: Cambridge University Press, 2005): 142–71; Adrienne Asch and David Wasserman, "Where is the Sin in Synecdoche? Prenatal Testing and the Parent-Child Relationship," in Wasserman, Bickenbach, and Wachbroit, *Quality of Life and Human Difference*: 172–216; and Dan Brock, "Is Selection of Children Wrong?" in Julian Savulescu and Nick Bostrom (eds.), *Human Enhancement* (Oxford: Oxford University Press, 2009): 251–76.

10.   Adrienne Asch, "Reproductive Technology and Disability," in Sherrill Cohen and Nadine Taub (eds.), *Reproductive Laws for the 1990s* (Clifton, NJ: Humana, 1989), p. 81.

11.   Marsha Saxton, "Disability Rights and Selective Abortion," in Rickie Solinger (ed.), *Abortion Wars* (Berkeley: University of California Press, 1997), p. 391.

12.   See, e.g., Asch and Wasserman, "Where is the Sin in Synecdoche?"

13.   This point is developed in Nelson, "Prenatal Diagnosis, Personal Identity, and Disability."

14.   For a classic work that develops this idea, see R. M. Hare, *The Language of Morals* (Oxford: Oxford University Press, 1952).

15.   A notable challenge to the moral acceptability of 2b comes from David Wasserman and Adrienne Asch in several of their writings (see, e.g., "Where is the Sin in Synecdoche?"). In their view, prospective parents *who have decided to become parents* (the qualification is important because the authors support abortion rights) should meet a standard of "unconditional welcome" in their attitudes and decisions regarding their children—a standard that is breeched when parents use PGD for negative selection. At the end of the argumentative day, however, Wasserman and Asch regard unconditional welcome as a moral ideal rather than an obligation. I am open to the possibility that the standard represents a moral ideal—at least, if it allows for certain exceptions—while noting that the assertion of this ideal is consistent with the claim that 2b is morally appropriate: To prefer not to have a child with a particular substantial disability could be morally acceptable even if not ideal.

16.   See, e.g., Union of the Physically Impaired Against Segregation, *Fundamental Principles of Disability* (London: UPIAS, 1976) and Ron Amundson, "Disability, Ideology, and Quality of Life: A Bias in Biomedical Ethics," in Wasserman et al., *Quality of Life and Human Difference*: 101–24.

17.   These models are helpfully discussed in Wasserman et al., *Quality of Life and Human Difference*, pp. 12–13.

18.   Jonathan Glover, *Choosing Children* (Oxford: Clarendon, 2006), p. 9.

19.   See, especially, Jeremy Bentham, *An Introduction to the Principles of Morals and Legislation* (1789).

20.   See, e.g., A. J. Ayer, "The Principle of Utility," in *Philosophical Essays* (London: Macmillan, 1954): 250–70.

21.   See, especially, James Griffin, *Well-Being* (Oxford: Clarendon, 1986).

22. See, e.g., Martha Nussbaum, *Women and Human Development* (Cambridge: Cambridge University Press, 2000). For an influential early work, see Amartya Sen, "Well-being, Agency, and Freedom," *Journal of Philosophy* 82 (1985): 169–221.

23. David Wasserman, "Philosophical Issues in the Definition and Social Response to Disability," in Gary Albrecht, Katherine Seelman, and Michael Bury (eds.), *Handbook of Disability Studies* (London: Sage, 2001), p. 230.

24. Some objective theorists construe intrinsically valuable functionings in a broader way that may appear to create more conceptual space for the idea that disabilities, even substantial ones, need not lower well-being. For example, rather than claiming that each of the five major senses is a component of well-being so that blindness entails an inherent prudential loss, one might hold that the relevant form of functioning is rich sensory experience, which a blind person may have through hearing and touch; rather than claiming that being able to use one's legs is a component of well-being, one might claim that being able to move around at will is the relevant capability. This is essentially the approach taken by Nussbaum (see *Women and Human Development*, pp. 78–79), whose list of central human capabilities has evolved over the years. But inasmuch as species-typical functioning includes the use of all the major senses and use of one's legs, it seems more consistent with the spirit of objective approaches to hold that blindness and paraplegia are inherently inimical to well-being even if neither, on its own, precludes a high overall quality of life. In any case, the objective theorist must surely judge that being thoroughly deprived of rich sensory experience or of the ability to move around at will is inimical to well-being—independently of effects on the individual's happiness. There are limits to how flexible an objective account can be.

25. For a good discussion, see Elizabeth Barnes, "Disability, Minority, and Difference," *Journal of Applied Philosophy* 26 (2009): 337–55, esp. 341–42.

26. See Robert Nozick's experience machine thought-experiment (*Anarchy, State and Utopia* [New York: Basic, 1974], pp. 42–45.

27. This suggestion and the one that follows come from L. W. Sumner, *Welfare, Happiness, and Ethics* (Oxford: Clarendon, 1996). With the third suggestion, I part ways with Sumner's account of well-being.

28. A full development of this theory will need to explain how to assess the well-being of individuals whose mental lives are less sophisticated than those of persons who can (1) have or fail to have a more or less accurate understanding of their circumstances and (2) judge how their overall lives are going. Perhaps my dog is well-off just to the extent that his subjective quality of life, or quality of experience, is high.

29. Wasserman makes roughly the same point ("Philosophical Issues in the Definition and Social Response to Disability," pp. 232–33).

30. In her valuable discussion, Barnes argues that disabilities (1) make life harder for those who have them and in that way constitute "local harms"—harms in relation to one area of an individual's life—but (2) cannot be expected to entail an overall lowering of the individual's well-being because of the way

in which individuals so often find meaning and special opportunities in the wake of particular hardships ("Disability, Minority, and Difference").

31. See Nicholas Wade, "A Decade Later, Genetic Map Yields Few Cures," *The New York Times* (June 13, 2010): A1, and Bijal Trivedi, Michael Le Page, and Peter Aldous, "The Genome—10 Years On," *New Scientist* (June 19, 2010): 30–37.

32. Green, *Babies by Design*, pp. 56–57.

33. Saul Kripke, *Naming and Necessity* (Cambridge, MA: Harvard University Press, 1980), p. 112.

34. *The Girl Who Played with Fire* (2009), directed by Daniel Afredson; based on Stieg Larsson's book *Flickan Som Lekte Med Elden* (Stockholm: Norstedts, 2006).

35. Whereas the concept of numerical identity was introduced in chap. 2 as the relation a thing has to itself in being one and the same individual *over time*, despite change, it is also the relation a thing has to itself in being one and the same individual *across "possible worlds" or possible situations*, despite qualitative differences. Here we are concerned with the "trans-world" dimension of numerical identity. We will also be concerned in this section with the cross-temporal dimension.

36. I am not contending that *no* conceivable change to a human organism would be identity-affecting. If a fetus, or a full-grown person, were changed so dramatically that a completely different kind of creature such as (what appeared to be) a fish or a plant were the result, we might have excellent grounds for asserting that the original human being was put out of existence and replaced with something else. But these are not the sorts of changes that we would consider in the name of PGT or PGE. Even the relatively far-reaching changes imagined in the thought-experiments about post-humans and post-persons in chap. 3 would not be identity-affecting. These changes were imagined to be relatively gradual, accruing over many generations.

37. See, e.g., Walter Glannon, *Genes and Future People* (Boulder, CO: Westview, 2001), pp. 81–82.

38. Noam Zohar, "Prospects for 'Genetic Therapy'—Can a Person Benefit from Being Altered?" *Bioethics* 5 (1991), p. 275.

39. Ibid, p. 283.

40. Jeffrey Kahn, "Genetic Harm: Bitten by the Body that Keeps You?" *Bioethics* 5 (1991), p. 299. Kahn articulates this reasoning without endorsing it.

41. See, e.g., Council on Ethical and Judicial Affairs, American Medical Association, "Genetic Engineering" (Opinion 2.13), in *Code of Medical Ethics* (Chicago: AMA, 2002).

42. Cf. John Harris, *Enhancing Evolution* (Princeton: Princeton University Press, 2007), p. 34.

43. *Babies by Design*, pp. 62–63.

44. See, e.g., John Robertson, *Children of Choice* (Princeton, NJ: Princeton University Press, 1994).

45. Joel Feinberg, "The Child's Right to an Open Future," in William Aiken and Hugh LaFollette (eds.), *Whose Child?* (Totowa, NJ: Rowman & Littlefield, 1980).

46. Buchanan et al., *From Chance to Choice*, p. 170.

47. Exemplifying such concerns are Dena Davis, *Genetic Dilemmas* (New York: Routlege, 2000) and Jurgen Habermas, *The Future of Human Nature* (Cambridge: Polity, 2003), pp. 61–63.

48. Cf. Green, *Babies by Design*, p. 127.

49. See, e.g., Andy Coghlan, "'Editing' Fixes Disease Gene," *New Scientist* (July 12, 2003): 3; T. Cathomen and M. D. Weitzman, "Gene Repair: Pointing the Finger at Genetic Disease," *Gene Therapy* 12 (2005): 1415–16; and Fyodor Urnov et al., "Highly Efficient Endogenous Human Gene Correction Using Designed Zinc-Finger Nucleases," *Nature* 435 (June 2, 2005): 646–51.

50. Michael Sandel, *The Case Against Perfection* (Cambridge, MA: Harvard University Press, 2007), p. 85

51. Cf. Green, *Babies by Design*, p. 225.

5

Bearing Children in Wrongful Life Cases

Tay-Sachs disease (TSD) is a fatal genetic disorder that causes large quantities of a fatty substance to build up in one's tissues and neurons. The disease is caused by deficiency of an enzyme, beta-hexosaminidase A, which catalyzes the breakdown of acidic fatty materials. Although rare forms of TSD can have a later onset, in its most common form the disorder affects its victims in infancy. After a few months of apparent normalcy, TSD infants begin a relentless decline in mental and physical abilities. They become blind, deaf, and unable to swallow. Their muscles atrophy, and paralysis gradually sets in. Other symptoms include dementia, seizures, and an increased startle reflex in response to noise. There is no treatment for TSD. For a while after onset of symptoms, seizures can be controlled with medicines. The prognosis, though, is extremely poor: Children usually die by age 4 from recurring infection.

Genetic carriers of TSD and affected individuals can be identified by a simple blood test that measures activity of the crucial protein. At especially high risk are people of East European descent and Ashkenazi Jews. Both parents must carry mutations in the *HEXA* gene to have an affected child, so each pregnancy poses a 25 percent risk of this calamity. Prenatal genetic diagnosis for this recessive genetic disorder is widely available.

Lesch-Nyhan syndrome (LNS) is a genetic disorder that is caused when deficiency of an enzyme, with the intimidating name of hypoxanthine-guanine phosphoribosyltransferase, allows the build-up of uric acid in body fluids. Symptoms that appear in the first year of life include severe gout, kidney stones and dysfunction, bladder stones, arthritis, poor muscle control, and moderate mental retardation. In the second year, self-mutilating behaviors such as lip biting, finger biting, and head banging appear. Neurological symptoms include facial grimacing, involuntary flailing and writhing, and repetitive movements such as those associated with Huntington's disease. Most affected individuals are unable to walk. There is no treatment for LNS, but some neurological symptoms can be alleviated with medications. Affected individuals usually die from renal failure in their first or second decade.

A recessive disorder, LNS is caused by mutations of the *HPRT 1* gene on the X chromosome. Thus, with very rare exceptions, only mothers pass on the disorder and only sons are affected. A daughter—inheriting two X chromosomes—cannot get the disease unless both parents are carriers, an extremely unlikely circumstance. In the more likely event that she inherits one mutated variant of the *HPRT* gene, the other, normal variant of the gene will permit more or less normal enzyme function. By contrast, a son who receives his only X chromosome from his carrier mother (his father contributing a Y chromosome to any son) has no second, normal variant of the relevant gene to permit healthy enzyme function. There are tests for carriers of LNS as well as prenatal tests for affected individuals.[1]

TSD and LNS impose terrible suffering and dysfunction on their victims. The life expectancy of affected individuals is very short. If the concept of wrongful life has any application, it presumably gets traction with these two disorders. The basic idea of wrongful life is that some diseases and perhaps some circumstances (e.g., slavery in especially brutal conditions) are so awful for the affected individuals that their lives are not worth living; moreover, knowingly to allow children to be born with such conditions or in such circumstances is to wrong them grievously. This idea compels us to consider whether, in creating children through procreation, we can wrong them.

It may seem obvious that to procreate, knowing that one's child will have TSD or LNS, wrongs the child by culpably harming her. The same sense of obviousness may accompany cases in which parents (or their doctors) did not know that their child would be affected but should have known or, in view of their carrier status or membership in a high-risk group, should have found out with testing. But, as courts began to realize by the 1970s, the basis of such a claim—that in such cases the affected child is wronged by being harmed—is far from clear.

Typically, in legal cases charging wrongful life, a congenitally impaired individual sues a physician for negligently "causing" him to be born.[2] Although our discussion will focus on the ethical issues attending parental decisions to bear a child, the same difficult conceptual issues arise whether it is a doctor's or a parent's liability that is in question and whether that liability is legal or ethical. Suppose a physician neglects to inform her pregnant patient that the patient's bout of rubella poses major risks to her fetus, which is later born deaf, blind, mute, and retarded. On behalf of the affected individual, a lawyer alleges that the physician was negligent in failing to inform the pregnant woman, who would have terminated the pregnancy and prevented great suffering to a child. A successful lawsuit would demonstrate that the physician had a duty to the plaintiff to provide sufficiently good care, that she failed to meet this duty, and that this failure caused an injury to the plaintiff.

But was there really any injury—any harm—to the child in bringing her into existence? The concept of harm is generally understood to be comparative and, in cases of bringing individuals into being, it is unclear whether there is an appropriate baseline for comparison. To say that A harmed B is generally understood as meaning that A caused B to be worse off in some way. A might have caused B to be worse off than he was beforehand (a historical conception of harm) or A might have caused B to be worse off than B would have been in the absence of A's intervention or culpable omission (a counterfactual conception of harm). Usually, both conceptions apply and converge. For example, if I am happily reading a book when you hurl a brick at my head, causing me great suffering and brain damage, then you have made me worse off than I was beforehand and worse off than I would have been had you refrained from assaulting me.

What is puzzling about charges of wrongful life, according to many commentators, is that neither the historical nor the counterfactual conception of harm seems to apply. If the alternative to the wrongful life is nonexistence, against what baseline can a harm be identified? Nonexistence is not a state of an individual, but rather the fact that there is no individual. So how can we say that bringing the child into existence—or failing to end her existence with abortion—made her worse off? Worse off than what? How could she have been better off?

This chapter will explore the ethics of wrongful life cases with considerable attention to conceptual issues that bear on the ethical issues. The chapter's two major sections will address the following questions. First, is it ever wrong to bring someone into being? If so, how can we coherently explain the nature of the wrong? Second, in view of the fact that human life always entails harms—to which no one consents before being brought into being—might it always be wrong to bear children? Are ordinary cases of childbearing more similar to those involving TSD or LNS than we commonly believe? In the concluding reflections, we will begin to consider how we can distinguish impermissible from permissible instances of procreation, setting the stage for Chapter 6.

MAKING SENSE OF WRONGFUL LIFE

The claim of wrongful life is the claim that bringing a child into being when it is known, or should be known, that the child is likely to have a certain condition wrongs the child. Usually, it is asserted that the child is wronged in being harmed. Is it intelligible to claim that one can be harmed by being brought into existence? Alternatively, if the child is not harmed by being brought into being, how can she be wronged?

Some individuals, perhaps on the basis of religious convictions, maintain that human life is so precious that any human life, regardless of its quality, is valuable to the individual living that life. All human lives are worth living. A realistic appreciation of what TSD and LNS involve puts any such optimistic contention into serious doubt. These two conditions—and no doubt some others—impose so much suffering and dysfunction on their victims, with so little prospect for compensating benefit, that it seems deeply implausible to claim that lives characterized by these conditions are worth living. I emphatically do not claim that these lives lack moral importance or that the individuals in question lack moral status. The present claim is not moral but prudential, addressing the interests of individuals afflicted with these conditions.

One might accept the claim that lives characterized by such conditions as TSD and LNS are not worth living without holding that being brought into existence with such a condition harms an individual. After all, one might claim that being brought into existence never harms or benefits anyone—on the grounds that existence cannot be compared with an alternative state of an individual. Such a comparison, the present reasoning continues, would be necessary to justify the idea that existence made one better off or worse off than one was before or would have been otherwise. Returning to our cases, while life with TSD or LNS clearly does not benefit one, perhaps it does not harm one either insofar as there was no other state that the individual ever was or could have been in. Nonexistence, again, is not a state of an individual, but rather the lack of an individual.

Now, those who believe in an afterlife can claim that death by abortion would be better than continued life, death being an alternative state that the individual can be in.[3] But they cannot claim that nonexistence (never existing) is a possible state that represents an alternative to being conceived in the first place. Moreover, their claim that failure to abort can constitute harm rests on the deeply contentious—some would say irrational—assumption of an afterlife. For the remainder of this discussion, I will ignore the possible assumption of an afterlife.

If nonexistence is not a state of an individual, can coming into existence—whose only alternative is nonexistence—be a harm? Some have argued that it can. One approach is to define harm normatively. For example, "a person is harmed at time T in respect R if his condition regarding R is worse than it should have been at time T."[4] But reference to the condition one should have been in implies that there is, in fact, another condition one could have been in—which is not the case if nonexistence is the only alternative. A more promising approach is to define harm noncomparatively by identifying general conditions that constitute harmful states. For example, "[a]n action harms a person if the action causes pain, early death, bodily damage, or deformity to her. . . ."[5]

Other approaches, while accepting that there is no harm to the victim in wrongful life cases, assert that the victim is nevertheless wronged. One strategy is to argue that in the cases under consideration, life with a terrible condition can be compared with nonexistence even though the latter is not a state one can be in. Joel Feinberg, for example, adduces this thought-experiment: God offers a dying person a choice between permanent extinction (nonexistence, not an afterlife) and reincarnation with TSD or a similarly awful disease. The more sensible choice, Feinberg plausibly claims, is nonexistence, showing that in a sense we can compare that option with that of a particular life.[6] Even though nonexistence is not a state, we might assign it a neutral value, contrasting it with the negative value of a life of terrible quality.

Another strategy capitalizes on comparisons between existence and nonexistence in the context of end-of-life decisions. We sometimes judge that it would be better for someone with terrible afflictions and no reasonable prospect of recovery to die earlier rather than later. This implies that the shorter life, considered as a whole, is better for him than the longer life, considered as a whole, providing a possible basis for saying that the victim is wronged in wrongful life cases.[7] But this approach only illuminates cases in which the charge of wrong applies to a failure to abort rather than the act of conceiving. Only in these cases can we compare two lives (one extremely short, in utero, the other extending past birth) of different duration.

A distinct approach is to argue that one can be wronged by being brought into being when one's life is noncomparatively bad.[8] Such lives are inherently bad for the subject in that whatever good they contain does not compensate for the bad; these lives are not judged bad by comparison to some other state one could have been in. One might claim that there is a right not to be conceived, or born, into a life that would predictably be bad in this noncomparative sense, but the rights-claim is not essential to the argument. What is centrally at issue is whether a claim of wrongdoing in wrongful life cases can be coherently supported.

At this point we have identified several fairly promising strategies for explaining how it is possible, in wrongful life cases, that the victim has been wronged. One possibility is that the victim was harmed in a noncomparative sense of harm. A disadvantage of this approach is that it rests on a nonstandard conception of harm and is therefore only as strong as the defense of that controversial conception (which will be taken up in Chapter 6). Other possibilities involve the idea that, although not harmed, the victim was wronged. We can remain neutral on the question of whether the nonstandard conception of harm is viable, and say that the other strategies share the idea that the victim was wronged whether or not she was harmed. She might have been wronged by being brought into existence in a state worse than the neutral value we can assign to nonexistence. Alternatively, the victim might have been wronged by not being aborted insofar as a very short life in utero would have been prudentially preferable to a much longer life with the debilitating condition. Finally, she might have been wronged by being created in a circumstance that was noncomparatively bad for her, the good in her life not compensating for the bad. Being unaware of any significant objection to this last claim, I find this strategy especially promising. In view of several promising strategies, especially the last one, I assume that the claim of wrongful life is perfectly intelligible. One can be wronged by being brought into existence.

MIGHT IT ALWAYS BE WRONG TO BRING SOMEONE INTO EXISTENCE?

It is one thing to contend that an individual can be wronged by being brought into existence. It is quite another to claim that one is always wronged by being brought into existence. This second claim contradicts the nearly universal assumption that it is morally permissible, often if not always, to bear children. The second claim may seem crazy. Yet substantial arguments can be adduced in its support.

Consider that all human lives contain harms. To be more precise and cautious, maybe we should say that all human lives that feature consciousness include harms. Arguably, a presentient fetus that is aborted is not harmed by death (see the discussion of this controversy in Chapter 2), and perhaps one who is born yet lives her entire life in a coma is harmed by neither death nor disability. What is indisputable is that virtually every human being who is born will encounter harm. To become sentient or conscious is to become exposed to harm. This means that the choice to bring someone into existence and into postnatal life (virtually) guarantees that the individual will suffer harms. Among those harms, most likely, will be the trauma associated with confronting one's own mortality. In the majority of cases in which death itself is properly regarded as a harm, as opposed to a blessing or a neutral event, one will incur the harm of death as well. In any case, one will also experience pain, disappointment, hurt feelings, and fear, no doubt at least some injuries, sickness, and other commonly incurred varieties of harm.

To be sure, most human lives also include substantial benefits, and one might think that these benefits typically compensate for the inevitable harms. But no one who is brought into being consents in advance to the overall life-package that includes future harms along with benefits. This is important because one might reasonably judge that it is wrong, or at least morally problematic, to harm an individual—or expose her to inevitable harm—without her consent, in order to benefit her. Relatedly, we tend to think it is more important, morally, not to harm others than it is to benefit them, at least in the absence of special circumstances (e.g., a contractual arrangement that demands some benefit while tolerating the risk of harm). For these reasons, one might seriously maintain that it is always wrong, or at least morally problematic, to bear children. The two most significant cases for such a pessimistic view have been developed by David Benatar and Seana Shiffrin, whose central arguments we will address in turn.[9]

Benatar's Challenge to Procreative Prerogatives

Most of us believe that even if some procreative decisions involve cases of wrongful life, most do not. We believe this at least in part because we believe that most human lives, while containing harms, also contain benefits sufficient to compensate for the harms, making those lives worth living. Benatar rejects this reasoning for several reasons.

ON "A LIFE WORTH LIVING"

First, Benatar contends, the argument fails to distinguish between two senses of "a life worth living": (1) a life worth starting and (2) a life worth continuing.[10] A person might judge that the benefits of his life compensate for the harms and that his life is for that reason worth continuing. That a life includes benefits that are sufficient—in the eyes of the one living the life—to compensate for the harms may seem an appropriate standard for judging that one's life is worth continuing. But we cannot straightforwardly infer that most cases of coming to be are not cases of wrongful life, because we cannot simply assume that an appropriate standard for a life worth continuing is also an appropriate standard for a life worth starting. Indeed, Benatar rejects this assumption. "For instance," he contends, "while most people think that living life without a limb does not make life so bad that it is worth ending, most (of the same) people also think that it is better not to bring into existence somebody who will lack a limb. We require stronger justification for ending a life than for not starting one."[11]

If Benatar is correct, then the distinction between the two senses of "a life worth living" may provide crucial support for his overall view. But I am not persuaded that the distinction is significant. Why should it matter whether one already exists when the question of whether one's life is worth living is raised? What is the basis for there being two standards rather than one? If a life is worth continuing, how could it not have been worth starting—considering that a necessary condition for continuing the life is having started it?

One possible reply appeals to the idea of completing projects that are already underway.[12] Sometimes it is worth finishing a project that one has begun and invested oneself in, even though it was not worth starting the project in the first place. One might feel that it was misguided to embark on the book one is writing—it would have been better to write a different book or do something entirely different with one's time—yet it would be a waste of all the effort that has gone into the present book not to complete it. One might even think of life as a whole as a project one invests in. This might justify the claim that a life that was not worth starting might nevertheless be worth continuing.

This reply is unpersuasive. The plausibility of examples such as the one about book-writing turns on a comparison between the prospect of completing one's current project and that of doing something else. If one never exists, there is no prospect of one's doing anything at all. If, instead of focusing on particular projects, we consider life as a whole as a project, the very possibility of investing in the life and finding it worthy of continuation represents an opportunity, not merely a burden. If creating a new life in such and such circumstances would appear to involve a strong chance that the person living it will value its continuation, that suggests—presumptively, not conclusively—that to start that life was good for that individual (assuming it makes sense to speak of one's coming into existence as a benefit or a harm for that individual). The life, presumably, was worth starting and not just continuing.

Another possible argument for the importance of the worth starting/worth continuing distinction appeals to the attractive idea that an already-existing person has some say in whether her life is worth living. Since most of us value our own lives, the argument goes, this fact generally enlarges the value of lives already underway (once their subjects can engage in prudential evaluation). Accordingly, the justification for ending a person's life would have to be stronger than the justification for not starting a human life. Hence two standards.

As it happens, Benatar is in no position to advance this argument. That is because he rejects prudential self-evaluation—which, in his view, is distorted by several pervasive psychological phenomena—as a significant factor in determining how well one's life is going.[13] The important issue, though, is not whether Benatar can advance this reply, but whether it is a persuasive reply. I doubt that it is. I strongly agree that an existing person has some say in whether his life is worth living. Because most of us value our lives, this implies that the value of a person's life is increased by his valuing it. Why, then, does that not mean that one's life is more valuable once one begins to value it, with the consequence that a life may become worth continuing even though it was not worth starting? Precisely because we know that most people value their own lives and prefer to continue them rather than die. Where one has reasonable grounds for predicting that an individual to be brought into existence will, like most people, come to appreciate her life, this consideration should be factored into a judgment as to whether the life is worth starting. To start the life is to have the opportunity to have a life that one values. It is not merely to be burdened with a mixed bag to which one did not consent.

I doubt that there is a solid basis for positing different standards for whether a life is worth starting and whether it is worth continuing. How, then, can one explain the point that "while most people think that living life without a limb does not make life so bad that it is worth ending, most (of the same) people also think that it is better not to bring into existence somebody who will lack a limb"? One can explain this point by distinguishing (1) the prudential question of whether a particular life is worth living from (2) the ethical question of whether it would be permissible not to start a particular life or to end a life in progress. One may hold, as I do, that a life featuring the absence of a limb is usually worth living while consistently maintaining that it may be morally best, or at least permissible, to decide not to bring into existence an individual who, foreseeably, will lack a limb. In Chapter 6, we will discuss why such a decision might be morally required or at least permissible. For now, it suffices to note that the judgment is an ethical one about reproductive decision-making, not a prudential judgment about whether the life in question is worth living. It would be naïve or dogmatic to assume that the only basis for such an ethical judgment is the prudential judgment. Other factors that may prove relevant (which we will discuss later) include (1) the value of reproductive freedom and (2) parental responsibilities to their offspring that go well beyond providing them a life worth living. My conclusion about the thesis that there should be different standards for a life worth starting and a life worth continuing is not that the thesis is clearly false, only that it is doubtful.

A Fundamental Asymmetry between Harm and Benefit?

We turn now to Benatar's main argument. According to Benatar, all cases of coming into existence are cases of harm. Earlier, we considered whether it makes sense to say that causing someone to exist in a wrongful life case harms that individual. We left that conceptual question open while concluding that there was sufficient reason to believe that causing someone to exist in such a case wrongs her. Let us here assume, at least for the sake of argument and convenience in engaging Benatar on his terms, that coming into being harms the one who comes into existence in wrongful life cases. Benatar's radical claim is that all cases of procreation are cases of this sort and are therefore cases of wrongful life.

Why think that everyone who comes into existence is thereby harmed? According to Benatar, all lives in the real world contain at least some harm. We granted this point earlier (with only a slight qualification, which we can ignore). But more needs to be said to explain why the inevitability of some harm in a life justifies the judgment that coming into existence is harmful all things considered. It may seem natural to think, on the contrary, that coming into existence can be either a net harm (harmful on balance even in view of anticipated benefits) or a net benefit (beneficial on balance even in view of anticipated harms). Why can't sufficient benefits in a life compensate for the harms?

The reason, Benatar argues, traces to a fundamental asymmetry between harm and benefit: The absence of harm is good, even if there is no subject of that good, yet the absence of benefit is not bad unless there is a subject for whom the absence constitutes a deprivation.[14] Benatar specifies that the absence of harm is good "when judged in terms of the interests of the person who would otherwise have existed" and, consequently, that "we have a strong moral reason, grounded in the interests of potential people, to avoid creating unhappy people."[15] Thus, he clearly means for the asserted fundamental asymmetry between harm and benefit to be grounded in individual-affecting reasons, which concern the interests of particular people or individuals (whether actual or possible). The asymmetry is not meant to be grounded in impersonal reasons, which concern the possibility of causing better or worse states of affairs irrespective of whether particular individuals are affected for better or worse. This is a problem, I suggest, because it is supremely doubtful that merely possible individuals have interests, there being no subject to have them. There are no free-floating interests; interests need a bearer, a subject. Only actual beings, I claim, have interests.[16]

One might wonder whether my insistence that only actual beings have interests is consistent with my acceptance of the thesis that there are cases of wrongful life. This thesis implies that certain individuals are wronged by being brought into existence. Before existing, were they not merely possible beings? If so, then it seems that, as possible beings, they had an interest in not being brought into a wrongful life. That suggests that possible beings, not only actual beings, can have interests.

I reject this reasoning and stand by my claim that only actual beings have interests. To speak of certain individuals' being wronged before they exist is to reify a mere possibility and treat it as a real entity—an individual (somehow existing?) prior to existing. This, it seems to me, is metaphysical nonsense that may be seductive only because ordinary language appears to permit reference to such nonentities with such phrases as "an individual prior to existing." If something does not yet exist, well, even that locution is misleading by appearing to refer to something; what we really have in mind is the absence of something. Note that, prior to conception, it is radically indeterminate who the possible person might be; prior to conception, there are millions of possibilities about who might be conceived.[17] Emphasizing the indeterminacy of "possible individuals" may make it easier to understand that they cannot be interest-bearing realities. Interests accrue when (or at least no sooner than) an individual comes into being—that is, when there is an actual being. Importantly, in cases of wrongful life there is an actual victim, the individual who is brought to term.

I have challenged Benatar's appeal to the putative interests of possible individuals. Would it strengthen Benatar's case for the asymmetry between harm and benefit if we reconstrued it as appealing not to particular individuals (including possible ones) but to impersonal value? The claim would be that absence of harm is impersonally good—being part of a better overall state of affairs than would exist in the presence of harm—while absence of benefit is not impersonally bad. But why accept this claim? After all, we can plausibly claim that absence of benefit is impersonally bad in the sense that it would be part of a less valuable overall state of affairs than would exist in the presence of benefit. So the proposed friendly revision of Benatar's argument in terms of impersonal value does not appear to strengthen it.

Benatar argues for the existence of a fundamental asymmetry between harm and benefit by contending that it best explains four other widely accepted asymmetries.[18] I paraphrase these four in italics and address them in turn.

A1. *There is a duty not to bring into being people who will predictably have terrible lives filled with suffering, but no duty to bring into being people who are likely to have good, happy lives.* I agree with this asserted asymmetry regarding procreative duties. But maybe, as Jeff McMahan argues, A1 is basic or fundamental, rather than resting on a more fundamental asymmetry such as the one Benatar defends (a general asymmetry between harm and benefit).[19] If so, one can accept A1 without accepting the more general asymmetry between harm and benefit. Another possibility, which may be attractive to those who find McMahan's thesis ad hoc, is that duties not to harm are generally much stronger than duties to benefit, a difference that arguably makes all the difference when we account for the importance of reproductive freedom. One way to specify this possibility is to assert the following principle: It is permissible (but never mandatory) to start a life only if that life is likely to be worth continuing.[20] On this principle, a predictably miserable life would be impermissible to start whereas a predictably good life would be permissible but not mandatory. So the plausible asymmetry regarding procreative duties, A1, is consistent with, but does not by itself favor, the fundamental asymmetry between harm and benefit championed by Benatar.

A2. *Whereas (i) it is of dubious intelligibility to give as a reason for having a child that the child will thereby be benefited, (ii) it makes sense to cite a potential child's interests as reason for not bringing a child into existence.* In response to clause (i), I suggest that it may very well make sense to say that coming into existence benefits the child who comes into existence, in which case one could intelligibly have a child for that child's sake. To be sure, one might doubt the coherence of claiming that coming into existence can benefit one: Prior to somebody's coming into being, there is no individual who can be benefited by coming to be (consistent with my claim that only actual beings have interests). Earlier, we noted that on a standard understanding of harm, one is harmed only if one is made worse off than one was beforehand or would have been otherwise. One who endorsed this conception of harm would make a parallel claim about benefit, which would require an independently existing subject who could be made better off. There being no such subject in the sorts of cases under consideration, one cannot, according to this reasoning, benefit by coming into existence. But this reasonable basis for rejecting the idea that one can be benefitted or harmed in coming into existence does not preclude other reasonable ways of viewing the matter. First, as noted earlier, one might adopt a normative conception of harm such that coming into existence in certain conditions constitutes harm; we could similarly adopt a normative conception of benefit. Second, although good sense requires us to deny that nonexistence is a harm or benefit—there being no actual subject with interests—we might reasonably hold that coming into existence with good prospects is a benefit (and that coming into existence with sufficiently bad prospects is a harm). Once one comes into being, there is an actual, identifiable subject who has interests—and we might judge that this determinate individual benefits from beginning a life with good prospects.[21] If this reasoning is correct, then one can, in a sense, have a child for that child's sake.

Contrary to clause (ii), I doubt that one can avoid having a child for that child's sake. If no child is brought into existence, then there is no actual individual who can benefit from the prospective parents' restraint. Again, only actual beings have interests. Now, if one does bring a child into being when one should not have done so in view of extremely poor prospects, then there is an identifiable victim of one's wrongful act: the actually existing child who has a terrible life. But it hardly follows from this, nor does it make sense in my judgment to claim, that some indeterminate, merely possible child benefits from a decision not to cause him to exist. (I do not deny that it can be in an actual fetus' interests not to be brought to term, but Benatar's claim applies even to merely possible, preconception "individuals.")

Suppose we focus on a case in which, say, a couple, both of whom are carriers for TSD, abstain from conceiving and procreating in order to avoid bringing into the world someone with this terrible disease. Can we not cogently say that they avoided having a child for the child's sake? Not really. Again, who is the child? There are an astronomical number of possible children who could have come into being had the couple conceived. We might miss this point by defining "the child" as "the one who would have come into being," but that is simply to cover up the indeterminacy of identity with a description; it is not to eliminate the indeterminacy inherent in the situation prior to conception.[22]

A3. Bringing someone into existence can be regretted for his sake, but not bringing someone into existence cannot be regretted for the possible individual's sake. Consistently with what I have argued, I agree. But, rather than explaining this conjunction of claims in terms of a fundamental asymmetry between harm and benefit, I explain it by reference to the fact that in the former case there is a subject of harm whereas in the latter case there is no such subject. Only actual beings have interests.

But can parents not be glad that they chose not to procreate when doing so would have created someone with a terrible disease? If so, can they not be happy for the sake of the individual, the merely possible individual, who was spared life with this condition?[23] Parents certainly can and should be glad in this circumstance, but—assuming they did not conceive—they cannot be glad for the sake of an individual who never exists because there is no such individual. Rather, they have reason to be glad because they avoided acting in a way that would have produced an actual individual who would suffer from the disease in question. Things would be different if the parents conceived and then aborted, for then there would have been an actual individual in whose interest it was not to be brought to term. Parents can terminate a pregnancy for the sake of the individual whose life is thereby shortened.

A4. We can rightly be sad about distant people who are known to languish, but not about possible people who would have flourished had they existed. Fair enough, but once again, I believe this claim is easily explained by the existence of actual victims in the first instance and the lack of any such victims in the second. Thus, like A1–A3, A4 does not favor the fundamental asymmetry between harm and benefit that Benatar champions in an effort to justify the radical thesis that existence has no advantage over, yet has disadvantages in comparison with, nonexistence. Nor is the asserted fundamental asymmetry particularly compelling on its face.

As an alternative to any picture incorporating the asymmetry Benatar champions, I recommend a picture that asserts the following:

> Regarding those who (actually) exist, the presence of benefit is good for them, and the presence of harm is bad for them. Regarding "those who never (actually) exist," the absence of benefit and the absence of harm are neither bad nor good for "them" because there are no such beings. Only actual beings have interests and can be benefited or harmed.

Note that it is consistent with this picture to assert the moral judgment that, generally speaking, it is more important to avoid harming than to benefit. This moral judgment may play a central role in explaining why we have an obligation not to procreate in wrongful life cases but no obligation to procreate where a child's prospects would be good, as captured in the principle stated earlier: It is permissible (but never mandatory) to start a life only if that life is likely to be worth continuing. But why, one may ask, may we ever procreate if it is more important, morally, to avoid harming—recall that all human lives involve harm—than to benefit? More will be said later in this chapter about considerations that may justify procreation, but for now it is worth noting that not harming may be generally more important than benefiting without the former being lexically prior to—that is, without having strict priority over—the latter. I would deny any such claim of lexical priority.

On the basis of the alleged fundamental asymmetry between harm and benefit, Benatar advances this remarkably strong thesis: "The harm of any pain [or any other harm] cannot be compensated for by even great amounts of pleasure [or any other benefit]. . . . "[24] Thus, on his view, the category of wrongful life encompasses all decisions to procreate regardless of the children's expected quality of life. Having rejected Benatar's central argument for this thoroughly pessimistic conclusion, we are well positioned to reject the conclusion—unless, that is, there are distinct, compelling arguments in its favor. To this possibility we now turn.

Shiffrin's Appeal to Unconsented Harms and Pure Benefits

Unlike Benatar, Shiffrin stops short of judging that all decisions to procreate are wrong. She contends, rather, that "because procreation involves a nonconsensual imposition of significant burdens, it is morally problematic and its imposer may justifiably be held responsible for its harmful results."[25] One might accept this thesis while holding that the value of procreative freedom, perhaps among other considerations, entails that at least some procreative acts, though morally problematic, are permissible, all things considered. Yet it is not difficult to see how the logic of her argument could lead one who accepts its premises to a thoroughly anti-procreation position like Benatar's.

Let me therefore present a Shiffrin-like argument. It is not exactly Shiffrin's argument because it arrives at a thoroughly anti-procreation conclusion. But it arrives at this conclusion on the strength of plausible premises, all endorsed or at least suggested by Shiffrin. I will italicize each step of the argument and discuss it before proceeding to the next step.

AN ANTI-PROCREATION ARGUMENT AND PRELIMINARY REFLECTIONS
1. *Coming into existence can be an overall benefit or harm.* We granted this assumption in replying to Benatar. In discussing the idea of wrongful life,

we saw that one might deny this assumption on the grounds that there is no independently existing individual who is benefitted or harmed by coming into being. But we also noted that, once one exists, there is an actual, identifiable individual who can be considered the subject of benefit or harm. Let us again, at least for the sake of argument, assume that the assumption is correct. Importantly, though, we should bear in mind that the assertion is that coming into existence can be an overall benefit or harm, not that it is in all cases.

2. *All human lives contain some substantial harms.* This seems undeniable. Even if a given person's life is an overall benefit to him, it will, as discussed earlier, inevitably contain some significant hardships, pain, and distress. (We can ignore possible exceptions involving those who never become conscious.)

3. *Although it is often permissible to cause an unconsented harm to avert a greater harm, it is impermissible to cause an unconsented (nontrivial) harm to procure "pure benefits"—goods that do not involve the removal or prevention of greater harm.* This claim is pivotal and merits careful attention.[26]

Consider a variation of a much-discussed case:

> Rescue. A man is trapped in a mangled car that apparently will explode within minutes. You alone can help. It appears that the only way of getting him out of the car will break his arm, but there is no time to discuss the matter. You pull him free, breaking his arm, and get him to safety before the car explodes.

In this case, you cause the (nontrivial) harm of breaking the man's arm, without his consent, in pursuing the only apparent way of averting a greater harm, his death. The man, who has no opportunity to consent, receives an overall benefit from your intervention. Your action is clearly permissible.

Now consider another case that also involves harming in an effort to confer an overall benefit:

> Gold manna.[27] An eccentric millionaire who lives on an island wants to give some money to inhabitants of a nearby island who are comfortably off but not rich. For various reasons, he cannot communicate with these islanders and has only one way of giving them money: by flying in his jet and dropping heavy gold cubes, each worth $1 million, near passers-by. He knows that doing so imposes a risk of injuring one or more of the islanders,

a harm he would prefer to avoid. But the only place where he can drop the cubes is very crowded, making significant (but nonlethal and impermanent) injury highly likely. Figuring that anyone who is injured is nevertheless better off for having gained $1 million, he proceeds. An inhabitant of the island suffers a broken arm in receiving her gold manna.

In this case, harm is imposed in a successful effort to confer an overall benefit on someone. But the specific benefit conferred, making someone $1 million richer, is a pure benefit; it does not involve averting a greater harm. And, of course, the islanders receiving the manna do not consent to the injury-risking but lucrative scheme. The fact that the millionaire imposes unconsented (nontrivial) harm in an effort to confer pure benefits helps to explain why his conduct is deeply troubling and perhaps impermissible.

4. *It does not harm a merely possible individual not to bring her into existence.* This assumption seems correct. It is supported by my earlier argument for the thesis that only actual individuals have interests.

5. *To procreate is to cause unconsented (nontrivial) harm to procure pure benefits.* Because human lives inevitably contain substantial harms, it may seem clear that to procreate is to cause harm to the individual created. Is "cause" quite the right word here, though? One who accepts the general spirit of this claim might prefer the term "impose." If so, premise 3 could be revised with a parallel substitution of "impose" for "cause." In any case, it cannot be claimed that causing or imposing the harm associated with human life is justified by averting a greater harm to the individual who is created, because, as just granted in 4, it would not harm a merely possible individual not to bring her into existence. Among justifications for procreation that appeal to the interests of the created individual, the only one that makes sense is an appeal to pure benefits: The individual brought into existence is likely to have an overall good life. So the italicized claim, one might hold, is justified—not because those who procreate are necessarily motivated by a desire to benefit their child, but because this is the strongest possible justification that appeals to the interests of the harmed individual, the child.

Therefore: 6. *To procreate is impermissible.* This thoroughly anti-procreation conclusion follows from the preceding claim and the earlier claim that it is impermissible to cause or impose unconsented (nontrivial) harm in order to procure pure benefits. The logic of this anti-natalist argument is clear. The argument is surprisingly compelling considering the incredible conclusion it supports. But is it really always wrong to bring children into the world? Or is the argument unsound?

CRITIQUE AND REFLECTIONS ON A MODIFIED FORM OF THE ARGUMENT

I believe the argument is unsound. Specifically, I think premises 3 and 5 are mistaken.

Starting with premise 3, there is a problem in asserting that causing unconsented (nontrivial) harm for pure benefits is impermissible. Consideration of such cases as Rescue and Gold Manna motivate this claim, but it also motivates a more modest claim: To cause unconsented (nontrivial) harm for pure benefits is morally problematic or pro tanto impermissible. In other words, to cause such harm for pure benefits tends to be wrong—has a wrong-making characteristic—but may be permissible in some circumstances in view of other values at stake. As explained later, this is the claim I endorse.

Premise 5 claims that procreating involves causing or imposing unconsented (nontrivial) harm to procure pure benefits. I suggest that this claim is overgeneralized. The characterization of "causing or imposing" the relevant harm applies only to those cases in which the act of procreation is closely and predictably tied to the imposition of significant disadvantage such as a major disability or a substantial socioeconomic disadvantage such as severe, entrenched poverty. To have a child in such cases is to impose the harm or hardship in question. What I deny is that the inevitability of harm in human life makes it apt to characterize all cases of procreation as involving the causing or imposition of harm. In the vast array of cases in which procreation is not closely and predictably tied to the imposition of significant disadvantage, I suggest that the procreative act is better characterized as *exposing* a child to harm: There is no harm closely associated with procreation in those circumstances, yet we know there will be some significant harm in that child's life. The difference between imposing harm and exposing to harm is significant.

"Exposing a child to harm" may sound bad, but we faultlessly expose children to harm all the time, often as part of creating opportunities for great benefits. Parents who enroll their children in school expose them to any manner of possible harms: humiliation in class, despair at being dumped by friends, depression secondary to poor performance or social difficulties, emotional and physical bullying, minor physical harms during recess or gym class, sleep deprivation, illness contracted from other students, and so forth. Nor would it make much sense to say that the children consent to be so exposed, considering their immaturity during most of their primary and secondary school years. Now consider examples outside the educational context. Parents who allow their children to join the Boy Scouts or Girl Scouts, participate in team sports, walk alone to friends' houses or the mall, drive a car when they are old enough, ride in a car at any time, and so on expose their children to harm—typically without meaningful consent, yet often faultlessly. Sometimes the exposure to harm is inextricably connected to the creation of opportunities for substantial benefits. In this light, bringing a child into the world where the child has good prospects in life and is not expected to have some major disability or hardship is not much like dropping gold cubes where they can land on someone. It is more like dropping gold cubes in the knowledge that passersby will pick them up and, simply by becoming wealthier, face an increased likelihood of being robbed and the emotional anguish of deciding which family members or charities to give to.[28]

Let us now consider a revised formulation of premise 3: *3R. . . . it is impermissible to expose one, without one's consent, to (nontrivial) harm in order to procure pure benefits.* Premise 3R would apply to the many cases in which procreation exposes the created individuals to the harms of life rather than more directly causing or imposing substantial harm or hardship. As suggested by the examples and revised gold manna case of the previous paragraph, 3R is implausible. In particular, it is not impermissible to expose children to the harms of life. Indeed, only in a somewhat trivial sense is it even pro tanto wrong to do so: Where the exposure to harm is not egregious—as it would be if parents made a young kid take up competitive boxing or form friendships with drug pushers— expected benefits easily compensate for the pro tanto wrongness in many cases.

If we think of procreative acts as dividing into those involving the imposition of harm and those involving mere exposure to harm, we can distinguish two modifications or specifications of premise 3. One, as suggested earlier in response to 3's assertion of impermissibility, is this: ". . . it is pro tanto wrong to impose an unconsented (nontrivial) harm to procure pure benefits." This, again, is relevant to cases in which the procreative act is closely and predictably tied to major harms or hardships for the child. Paradigm wrongful life cases, in which life seems clearly not worth living (either starting or continuing), are among these cases. Indeed, in such cases there are so few benefits in prospect that the harms would clearly outweigh them, so that procreation here is not just pro tanto wrong but also all-things-considered wrong. But other sorts of cases fall under the scope of this principle: cases in which, say, the child will be born with a major disability yet the life is expected to be worth living. Procreation in these cases is pro tanto wrong, but it may sometimes be permissible, all things considered (as discussed in Chapter 6).

In those cases in which it is exposure to harm that is at issue, the relevant revision of 3 is this: ". . . it is pro tanto wrong to expose one to (nontrivial) harm, without one's consent, in order to procure pure benefits." But, as mentioned earlier, only in a trivial sense is it even pro tanto wrong to do so. Where the exposure to harm is not egregious, expected benefits frequently justify the possibility of harm.

At this point, we may summarily say the following:

- In paradigm wrongful life cases—in which the life in question would not be worth living—procreation is wrong;
- In other cases involving the imposition of harm, procreation is (strongly) pro tanto wrong;
- In cases involving only exposure to harm (at least where it is not egregious), procreation is (weakly) pro tanto wrong.

What sorts of moral considerations can serve to justify procreation in the second and third classes of cases despite its pro tanto wrongness?

Considerations That May Justify Procreation

I contend that two, and possibly three, considerations justify procreation in the instances in which it is justified: (1) procreative freedom, a central interest of prospective parents; (2) the interests of the child brought into being; and possibly (3) the impersonal value of bringing more net good into the world.

The case for the relevance of the first consideration rests on the reasonable assumption that the interests of those who wish to be parents count for something and that, among their interests, procreative freedom (procreative liberty, procreative autonomy) is especially important. The value of procreative freedom is widely invoked in reproductive ethics. In the words of John Robertson, a prominent spokesperson for reproductive prerogatives, "[p]rocreative liberty should enjoy presumptive primacy when conflicts about its exercise arise because control over whether one reproduces or not is central to personal identity, to dignity, and to the meaning of one's life."[29] Whether or not to have children, when and by what means to have them, how many to have, and similar choices are extremely important to us. These decisions greatly affect our narrative identity—for example, whether or not we become parents, what sort of family we have—and much of the shape of our lives. Few decisions seem as personal and far-reaching as reproductive decisions. That procreative freedom is very important seems too obvious to require further defense.

At the same time, we need to know whether the importance of procreative freedom can, by itself or in conjunction with other considerations, override pro tanto obligations not to (impose or expose to) harm. Robertson and many other scholars take the value of procreative freedom to have a sort of presumptive force. "Such a presumption," Robertson clarifies, ". . . means that those who would limit procreative choice have the burden of showing that the reproductive actions at issue would create such substantial harm that they could justifiably be limited."[30] But hardly any scholars who celebrate the value of procreative freedom have fully appreciated the fact that human procreation involves, even in the most benign cases, exposure to substantial harm.

Those who have appreciated this fact have generally assumed that, where a child's prospects are good, the particular benefits in the created life are likely to compensate for the particular harms, so that the imposition of or exposure to harm is justified by an overall benefit to the individual created. If so, then even if we regard the justifiable prerogatives of child-bearing as limited by the harm principle—roughly, the principle that we should not knowingly or negligently harm others—we can assert that this principle applies only where a child's life is expected to constitute an overall harm to her. This, according to the present reasoning, is not often the case, so the concept of wrongful life applies only to reproductive decisions that are especially irresponsible. The fact that all human lives involve some substantial harm is irrelevant. What is important is a potential child's overall life prospects.

Our reflections reveal that this congenial line of reasoning is, in many instances, insufficient to justify procreation. Where procreation involves merely exposing a child to harm, a justified expectation that the benefits of a child's life will outweigh the harms—in combination with the value of procreative freedom—is plausibly thought, in many cases, to overturn the relatively weak pro tanto wrongness of exposing the child to harm by causing her to exist; the examples provided earlier of parents' justifiably exposing their children to harm support this judgment. But consider cases that feature the expectation of a life worth living while imposing a major disability or other hardship. Procreation in these cases was judged to be strongly pro tanto wrong. Might procreation in all such cases be simply wrong, not just pro tanto wrong? Think of cases in which, say, parents know that any child they have will be blind. Supposing the parents cannot adopt, greatly want to have a child, and realistically expect that the child will have a good life despite blindness, is it obvious that neither procreative freedom nor any other consideration could justify their decision to have a blind child? I do not think so.

The most persuasive case that such a decision can sometimes be justified is a persuasive argument that imposing unconsented (nontrivial) harm is sometimes justified in pursuit of pure benefits. I believe this is correct. I submit that appropriate parenting features many cases of this sort. Sometimes parents make their children enter into endeavors whose pursuit guarantees such nontrivial harms as frustration, deep disappointment, loss of opportunities to do other things that are important to the children such as spending more time with friends or relaxing, and in some cases a high likelihood of physical pain and occasional injury. This is often the case when parents push a child to be an outstanding scholar, musician, or athlete. The sacrifices and risks required in these pursuits are generally motivated not by a desire to avoid greater harm—as if being less than outstanding were harmful—but by a desire for pure benefits: accomplishment, enhanced discipline and focus, greater self-esteem, glory, admission to a selective university, or whatever. To be sure, in many cases the parental push that guarantees some occurrence of harm is unjustified: The parents push too hard, they neglect their child's psychological health, or they leave him too few possibilities for the long-term future (see the discussion of the "right to an open future" in Chapter 4). But in many cases, I suggest, the parental push is morally permissible and even highly commendable: Likely harms are minimized (though they remain nontrivial), the prospect for personal reward is great, and the child's future possibilities are left reasonably open. I am fairly confident that the reader will agree with me on this point.[31]

Now consider another sort of case that involves imposing unconsented harm for pure benefits. Sometimes a government will force a property owner to move, whether she wants to or not, in order to permit the construction of roads, a dam, or some other source of pure benefit. Forcing a reluctant individual to move entails stress, frustration, the inconvenience of moving, and sometimes loss of certain advantages that are unique to the home she must vacate. This setback to the property owner's interests is a harm because she is, in several respects, made worse off than she was before the imposition and worse off than she would have been without it. Now, it is generally assumed that property owners forced to relocate are owed compensation. But, if they would still prefer not to move, the compensation simply counts as a form of pure benefit to them, part of an overall package of harm and benefit to which they did not consent. Those who believe that it is sometimes justified to require people to relocate in order to make possible certain benefits for the broader community seem to accept the idea that it is sometimes permissible to impose unconsented harm for the sake of pure benefits—here, primarily for the community. They should believe, a fortiori, that it is sometimes permissible to impose unconsented harm for the sake of pure benefits when the latter accrue primarily to the individual harmed.

We have found some support for the thesis that procreative freedom along with consideration of the created child's interests can sometimes justify bringing children into being even when a substantial harm or burden is imposed on them. But the case for this thesis is incomplete. More needs to be said about the child's interests as a source of justification.

In this vein, I appeal to what I call the "undeluded gladness factor": the fact that, among the enormous number of people who are glad to be alive (many of whom live with the challenge of a significant disability or socioeconomic disadvantage), many and perhaps most of them cannot rightly be regarded as basing their gladness on a deluded, inflated estimation of their own well-being. Benatar has developed an extensive argument that the typical human gladness to be alive and a strong preference to continue living are untrustworthy as bases for evaluating human well-being. His defense of this claim has several components and contains many good points, but here I will recapitulate neither his arguments nor my replies to them.[32] Consistent with the value theory defended in Chapter 4—and, I submit, any remotely plausible value theory—we must take seriously the fact that many people enjoy their lives, want them to continue (not just because they are afraid to commit suicide), and believe that they are going pretty well by standards appropriate for human beings. To be sure, it is possible to contend that such optimistic judgments are pervasively distorted by wishful thinking, irrelevant comparisons to others, and a biologically adaptive prejudice in favor of living and against self-destruction. But the more reasonable course, in my view, is to believe that many (not all) people who believe their lives are going well for them and are worth living are justified in thinking so.

Now, the importance of undeluded gladness about being alive concerns what it suggests about the interests of the individual who was brought into being. For it strongly suggests (1) that the individual's life is an overall benefit to him (an appeal to his well-being or quality of life), and (2) that he embraces the overall life-package of harms and benefits he was given despite never having had any opportunity to consent to it (an appeal to his will). The undeluded gladness factor helps us to appreciate that being brought into existence entails not only a burden but also an opportunity. This is the opportunity to have a life that one may well come to embrace and find worthwhile. These points suggest that the child's prospects and (once he exists) his interests are an important consideration that can play a justifying role in many cases of procreation, even where harm is imposed. In Chapter 6, we will we endeavor to formulate standards or criteria for justified procreation that do justice to the child's interests. In the meantime, it is worth noting that the undeluded gladness factor suggests one possible criterion, or at least a necessary condition, for permissible procreation: when prospective parents can make a reasonably confident, justified prediction that their child will come to enjoy and appreciate her life (without denial about her circumstances or other obvious distortions in her self-evaluation of well-being).

We have found that (1) procreative freedom and (2) a prospective child's good prospects (the realistic prospect for undeluded gladness and the good life it reflects) both help to justify some procreative choices despite their pro tanto impermissibility. In my view, a third factor might play a role in justifying those procreative acts that are permissible. Note that the two factors considered so far are individual-affecting, bearing on the interests of actual individuals. Procreative freedom is an important interest of individuals who are considering the possibility of having a child. A child's prospects, of course, concern her own future interests. The third possible factor, by contrast, is impersonal: the possibility of increasing the amount of net good in the world. The idea is simply that, by creating an individual who is likely to have a life that is, on balance, good for her—assuming there is not an offsetting amount of harm caused to others by her existence—parents make the world a slightly better place. Does this impersonal factor help to justify permissible instances of procreation?

One might doubt it. As noted earlier, whereas the likelihood that a child one could bring into existence would have a miserable life supports an obligation not to procreate, the likelihood that a child one could bear would have a good life does not support an obligation to procreate. This is the asymmetry regarding procreative duties. But perhaps the likelihood that one would have a happy, flourishing child provides a reason to procreate without creating an obligation. If, as seems plausible, we generally have stronger obligations not to harm than to benefit, we may have an impersonal moral reason to procreate when one's child's prospects would be good; but it may be a reason that, given the importance of procreative freedom, never amounts to an all-things-considered obligation to procreate. Perhaps. I will leave open the issue of whether, in addition to procreative freedom and the child's good prospects, the impersonal value of producing more net good in the world helps to justify some instances of procreation.

FURTHER REFLECTIONS AND CONCLUSIONS

In this chapter, we have examined the concept of wrongful life and two fundamental ethical issues associated with this concept. Regarding the question of whether there is such a thing as wrongful life, we answered affirmatively. Rather than adopting a single way of understanding the wrong in question, we noted several promising possibilities for understanding this wrong and assumed that at least the approach that appeals to the idea that some lives are noncomparatively bad for their subjects would survive critical scrutiny. In light of arguments developed by Benatar and Shiffrin, we then asked whether it might be the case that all procreative acts were cases of wrongful life. Acknowledging that Shiffrin had raised legitimate concerns about the relationship of procreating to harm—at least exposing children to harm, sometimes more directly imposing it—we went on to argue that many procreative acts could nevertheless be justified on the basis of procreative freedom, the realistic prospect of benefit to the child as suggested by the undeluded gladness factor, and, possibly, impersonal beneficence as well.

This conclusion leads us to the question of which procreative acts are justified. What are the criteria for permissible procreation? It is enormously difficult to say. As a start, we might highlight paradigm cases of wrongful life such as knowingly or negligently bringing into the world an individual with TSD or LNS. Obviously, permissible instances of procreation are not like these. As stated earlier, it is permissible to start a life only if it would likely be worth continuing. But few procreative decisions feature odds stacked so terribly against the individual to be created as they are in the paradigm wrongful life cases, and we can hardly assume that these are the only impermissible cases of procreation.

In the preceding section, we arrived at a necessary condition for permissible procreation: that there is good reason to expect that the individual to be created will come to appreciate and enjoy her life, feeling glad to be alive, without her judgment being deluded. This begins to specify the principle that we may start a life only if it is likely to be worth continuing. But, in order to distinguish impermissible from permissible acts of procreation, we need to know what conditions are necessary and jointly sufficient.

Here is one possible approach. We could argue, first, that cases of wrongful life are precisely those in which it is predictable that the individual to be created would have a life filled with suffering and dysfunction with negligible prospect for compensating satisfaction or meaning. Someone living such a life, if capable of evaluating and communicating about her life, would not (in the absence of severe delusion) express gladness about her life as a whole. We might then accept that all other lives, the vast majority, are lives worth living—or at least lives that we should presume are worth living. That is, only the paradigm wrongful life cases feature lives that are (presumably) not worth living—neither worth starting nor worth continuing. And the only wrongful life cases, the only circumstances in which it is wrong to procreate, are those in which the lives, predictably, would be of this sort.

This approach connects the concepts of wrongful life and a life worth living in an elegant, perspicuous way. But I am convinced that this approach is mistaken. As I will argue in the next chapter, parents generally owe their children much more than simply a life worth living. Irresponsible procreation covers far more instances than the paradigm wrongful life cases. Compared to the neat solution just sketched, the approach developed in the next chapter is more consonant with the insight that procreation involves at least exposure to—and often the imposition of—significant harms and is therefore a morally momentous decision.

NOTES

1. For information on these and other inheritable disorders, see Genetic Home Reference (http://ghr.nlm.nih.gov/conditions) and, for inheritable neurological disorders in particular, the National Institute of Neurological Disorders and Stroke Web site (www.ninds.nih.gov/disorders).
2. For a good introduction to the legal cases, see E. Haavi Morreim, "The Concept of Harm Reconceived: A Different Look at Wrongful Life," *Law and Philosophy* 7 (1998), pp. 4–10.

3. Of course, if they also hold that abortion is morally impermissible—as many who believe in an afterlife do believe—they will not claim that failure to abort wronged the individual who was born.

4. Morreim, "A Different Look at Wrongful Life," p. 23.

5. Elizabeth Harman, "Can We Harm and Benefit in Creating?" *Philosophical Perspectives* 18 (2004), p. 93.

6. "Wrongful Life and the Counterfactual Element in Harming," in Joel Feinberg, *Freedom and Fulfillment* (Princeton: Princeton University Press, 1992), pp. 3–36.

7. Allen Buchanan, Dan Brock, Norman Daniels, and Daniel Wikler, *From Chance to Choice* (Cambridge: Cambridge University Press, 2000), pp. 234–35.

8. Jeff McMahan, "Wrongful Life: Paradoxes in the Morality of Causing People to Exist," in Jules Coleman and Christopher Morris (eds.), *Rational Commitment and Social Justice* (Cambridge: Cambridge University Press, 1998), p. 215.

9. See Benatar, *Better Never to Have Been?* (Oxford: Oxford University Press, 2006) and Shiffrin, "Wrongful Life, Procreative Responsibility, and the Significance of Harm," *Legal Theory* 5 (1999): 117–48. The discussion of Benatar that follows draws significantly from my "Is it Wrong to Impose the Harms of Human Life? A Reply to Benatar," *Theoretical Medicine and Bioethics* 31 (2010), pp. 320–24.

10. *Better Never to Have Been*, pp. 22–23.

11. Ibid, p. 22.

12. Cf. David Velleman, "Persons in Prospect," *Philosophy and Public Affairs* 36 (3) (2008), p. 274.

13. *Better Never to Have Been*, chap. 3.

14. Ibid, p. 30. He states his thesis with reference to pain and pleasure, taking these to be clear instances of harm and benefit, respectively. To avoid misunderstanding, I prefer to use the more comprehensive categories of harm and benefit.

15. Ibid, pp. 31, 33.

16. Cf. Jeff McMahan, "Asymmetries in the Morality of Causing People to Exist," in Melinda Roberts and David Wasserman (eds.), *Harming Future Persons* (Dordrecht, Netherlands: Springer, 2009), p. 63. One might challenge my claim that only actual beings have interests on the grounds that future persons seem to have interests, providing a basis for our obligations to future generations not to be negligent with the environment and scarce resources. I disagree, though, that future persons *now* have interests and leave until Chapter 7 to explain the basis of our obligations to future generations.

17. Here I assume that "possible individuals" are not souls waiting in line to be conceived. If they were, then these individuals would already exist in immaterial form. I assume that there is no good reason to believe such a thing and much good reason not to.

18. *Better Never to Have Been*, pp. 32–35.

19. McMahan, *The Ethics of Killing* (New York: Oxford University Press, 2002), pp. 353–54.

20. Cf. Thaddeus Metz, "Are Lives Worth Creating?" *Philosophical Papers* 40 (2) (2011): 233–55.

21. Derek Parfit tentatively defends this thesis (*Reasons and Persons* [Oxford: Clarendon, 1984], Appendix G).

22. Moreover, whoever is conceived would most likely be disease-free. With two carriers of the disease gene, the odds that any given conception will produce a fetus with TSD is one in four (much too high to take the risk responsibly, unless the couple is prepared to abort, but less likely than the 75 percent chance of a normal pregnancy). This point does not apply in cases in which a terrible disability or circumstance is the more likely outcome, but the decisive point about radical indeterminacy remains.

23. Cf. Caspar Hare, "Voices from Another World: Must We Respect the Interests of People Who Do Not, and Will Never, Exist?" *Ethics* 117 (2007), p. 499.

24. *Better Never to Have Been*, p. 48.

25. "Wrongful Life, Procreative Responsibility, and the Significance of Harm," p. 139.

26. It also may be stronger than Shiffrin's view. Changing "impermissible" to "morally problematic" in (3) would clearly be faithful to what she argues, but her examples and discussion leave unclear why we should stop short of the stronger claim of impermissibility.

27. This is a variation of a case presented in Shiffrin, "Wrongful Life, Procreative Responsibility, and the Significance of Harm," p. 127.

28. Thanks to Frances Kamm, who suggested this analogy to me.

29. John Robertson, *Children of Choice* (Princeton: Princeton University Press, 1994), p. 24. For another good discussion, see Buchanan et al., *From Chance to Choice*, chap. 6.

30. *Children of Choice*, p. 24.

31. For any reader who is skeptical, I recommend the movie *Temple Grandin* (2010, directed by Mick Jackson). In this movie, which is based on a true story, Grandin's mother heavy-handedly pushes her autistic, socially low-functioning daughter to enter college, against her wishes, although it is very clear that doing so will entail considerable stress and psychological pain for Grandin. Here, I think, is a vivid case of a parent justifiably imposing significant, unconsented harm on her child in pursuit of pure benefits.

32. His case is developed in *Better Never to Have Been*, chap. 3. My reply is contained in "Is it Wrong to Impose the Harms of Human Life? A Reply to Benatar."

6

Bearing and Caring for Children with Disadvantage

It was argued in Chapter 5 that there are rare cases in which procreating is wrong because the resultant child's life predictably will not be worth living. These are the paradigm wrongful life cases. Are there other cases in which procreation is wrong because of the children's expected quality of life? Parents, it seems, owe their children much more than just a life worth living. What do parents owe their children? In what sorts of cases—beyond the paradigm wrongful life cases—is it wrong to procreate?

Approaching our questions from another angle, is there a moral right—or any significant moral prerogative—to bear children? If so, what is its basis? And what are its limits? Presumably, moral limits to procreative freedom are set, at least primarily, by what parents owe their children. It seems sensible that parents owe their children not just a life worth living, but certain resources and conditions that contribute to a *decent* human life. A special puzzle called *the nonidentity problem* arises, however, in cases in which parents cannot confer the resources and conditions they seemingly owe their children on *a particular child whom they bear*, a child who nevertheless has a life worth living. How to account for the apparent wrong of procreating in these cases, in view of the fact that the child owes his worthwhile existence to the procreative act in question? This chapter confronts these questions.

As in the previous chapter, the focus will be on procreation—consistent with the central theme of this book, creation ethics—as opposed to adoption, another way of having children. More specifically, the chapter will focus on procreation with the intention of *raising* the created child rather than giving her up for adoption. Since the prerogative to procreate is limited by what parents owe their children, the norms to be defended will be centrally concerned with morally adequate parenting. Thus they will primarily apply to what we may call *procreation plus parenting*. At the same time, they will also prove relevant to adoption insofar as what parents owe their children also sets limits on the moral prerogative to adopt. Someone who is highly likely to abuse any child he or she raises, for example, should not become a parent, whether through procreation or adoption.

Throughout the discussion, we will focus on cases featuring lives that are presumably worth living yet impose substantial disadvantage on the child brought into existence. The emphasis here is on *substantial* disadvantage. As discussed in Chapter 5, every human life involves pain, distress, loss, and misfortunate to some nontrivial degree. Every human life involves harm and burden. Here we will focus on cases in which the predictable harm or burden is large enough to provoke the question of whether it is right knowingly to bring into being someone who will endure the hardship—which may be a (nontrivial) disability such as blindness, deafness, or a missing limb or a life circumstance such as great poverty, parents who are themselves children, or slavery.

In addressing procreation that may impose substantial disadvantage on offspring, we will distinguish three kinds of procreative choice[1]:

1. *Same-individual choices*: Having a child with disadvantage versus having the same child without disadvantage;
2. *Different-number choices*: Having a child with disadvantage versus not having a child;
3. *Same-number choices*: Having a child with disadvantage or, by delaying conception or aborting and conceiving again, having a different child without disadvantage.

Different moral analyses will prove appropriate to the three kinds of procreative decision.

The remainder of the chapter begins with a section on what parents owe their children. In the next section, it is argued that in same-individual choices the importance of procreative freedom is outweighed in a relatively straightforward way by considerations of the child's interests. It is contended in the section that follows that procreative freedom carries greater weight with different-number choices than it does with same-individual and same-number choices.

Turning in the next section to same-number choices, we encounter the non-identity problem. A variety of strategies for resolving this problem are identified and appraised, and a solution is suggested. The final section recapitulates major findings from the previous sections, draws connections among them, sketches a view of wrongful disadvantage (a kind of wrongful life), and elicits implications for the ethics of procreating in a variety of circumstances in which prospective parents may find themselves.

WHAT PARENTS OWE THEIR CHILDREN: CONSTRAINTS ON PROCREATIVE FREEDOM

We begin with the assumption, defended in Chapter 5, that procreative freedom is an important value. As the discussion of wrongful life cases made clear, this important value is not absolute. According to some, procreative freedom may be limited in the name of protecting social values such as avoiding hurtful, demeaning messages to persons with disabilities (as discussed in Chapter 4) or in order to avoid disastrous overpopulation. In this discussion, we will focus on whatever limits to procreative freedom are justified by reference to the interests of prospective offspring. What do parents owe their children? Consistently with the case developed in Chapter 2 for the permissibility of abortion, the scope of "their children" in this discussion is limited to those offspring who are brought to term. The position to be developed implies that there is no *moral right* to procreate—where rights are understood as nearly absolute prerogatives or entitlements—but rather a significant, yet limited, *moral prerogative* to do so. Those who use rights language more promiscuously may articulate the same idea by stating that the right to procreate is significantly qualified or conditional.

We may distinguish several positions in response to the question of what parents owe their children. Consider first the view that what parents owe their children is (the likelihood of) *a worthwhile life*. Parents should not procreate when it appears unlikely that their offspring would have a life worth living, but in all other cases it is permissible to procreate.

One difficulty in assessing this worthwhile-life view arises from the fact that, as Jonathan Glover puts it, the idea of a life barely worth living is "a philosopher's abstraction" that is very difficult to specify.[2] We may be confident that cases of intentionally or negligently bearing children with Tay-Sachs disease[3] (TSD) or Lesch-Nyhan syndrome (LNS) fall short of the worthwhile-life standard, as discussed in Chapter 5. We might confidently add to the wrongful life category cases in which, say, a child will predictably be blind, deaf, profoundly retarded, and incapable of reaching adult age. But few cases are as bleak as this. On the other side of the imaginary line marking a worthwhile life, surely, are cases of mild mental retardation and cases of deafness. So there are some obvious cases on each side of the line. Between these two sets of easy cases, however, is a large grey area.

Notwithstanding this grey area, the worthwhile-life standard seems grossly inadequate. Imagine wealthy, healthy prospective parents who are in a position to offer their children excellent prospects in life but, out of pure self-indulgence, set very low parenting standards for themselves. They will make sure their children have shelter, something to eat at least a couple of times a day, and access to school, but the parents do not intend to spend very much time with them, encourage their personal development, or save any money for college. Nor do they intend to prevent their kids from watching television during most of their free time or experimenting with drugs at an early age. Even on the assumption that the children's lives will be predictably worth living, this degree of parental negligence seems extremely irresponsible—and to procreate with the intention, or likelihood, of parenting in this way seems wrong.

In this case, it is striking how much more than just a life worth living the parents could provide their children. Perhaps what parents owe their children is determined in part by what they *can* provide them. Maybe, for example, the fortunate parents just described owe their children enough in savings to enable a private university education whereas working-class parents do not owe this particular benefit to their children. While leaving space for some differences in what parents owe their children seems reasonable, there remains the question of what all parents owe their children.

Should we say that all parents owe their children *(1) worthwhile lives and (2) whatever other benefits they, in view of their circumstances, can provide them*? This proposal has several interesting consequences.

First, in addition to condemning the irresponsible, advantaged parents who can't be bothered to provide their children much more than a life worth living, since these parents would fail criterion (2), the proposal would judge all parents who provide less than they can for their children to have acted wrongly. That is too strict. While "providing the best for one's children" has an attractive ring, it sets an implausibly high standard—assuming it is taken literally and understood as a standard of parental duty rather than an ideal. As discussed in Chapter 4, parents cannot be expected always to do what literally *maximizes* their children's interests. Sometimes other legitimate interests—such as those of the parents themselves, particular communities, or charities—legitimately compete with children's interests, notwithstanding the extensive partiality towards one's children that is essential to good parenting.

Thus, rather than a standard of literally doing the best for one's children, it seems more sensible to hold that parents owe their children *(1) worthwhile lives (2) in which their basic needs (essential interests) are reasonably expected to be met and (3) doing more for them where the parents can without undue sacrifice.*

Two clarifications are in order. First, the second criterion stipulates that basic needs "are reasonably expected to be met" rather than "will be met" because parents often cannot guarantee that certain basic needs will, in fact, be met. For example, even a parent who provides a very safe environment for her child cannot guarantee that the child will not, through a bizarre sequence of events, be kidnapped and mistreated. Second, the concept of undue sacrifice in the third criterion is not elaborated, but an example may help to flesh out the idea. Suppose a child's basic needs will easily be met even if both parents work outside the home, yet the child would do a little better if one parent sacrificed his or her career. But both parents consider it essential to their flourishing to continue their careers. In this circumstance, reluctantly sacrificing his or her career would plausibly count as an undue sacrifice.

Returning to the two-part standard under consideration (see three paragraphs above), one of its implications is that where parents, given their circumstances, *cannot* do better for their children than provide them lives worth living, this provision is morally sufficient. One might judge that this is overly permissive: Children's basic needs, one might argue, constitute a non-negotiable baseline. But imagine prospective parents who seem capable of providing any child they have with a worthwhile life yet, due to circumstances beyond their control such as entrenched poverty and political oppression, cannot reasonably ensure that some of their child's basic needs will be met. To deny these individuals the opportunity to become parents may be to give too little weight to procreative freedom and to allow socioeconomic disadvantage too great a role in determining the prerogatives of parenthood. With this point in mind, one might judge that parents owe their children the following: *(1) worthwhile lives, (2) meeting whichever of the children's basic needs the parents can meet and (3) doing more for them where the parents can without undue sacrifice.*

But what if prospective parents cannot meet one or more basic needs of children, but only because of their own character or psychological constitution? Suppose a man cannot ensure any child he has a reasonable degree of physical safety because he has a compulsion to abuse children. If he can't eradicate this compulsion through psychotherapy or other means, he seems unfit to become a parent. Perhaps the good idea behind a willingness to tolerate exceptions to the rule that children's basic needs must be met is that it would be unfair to prospective parents to expect them to forego having children in precisely those cases in which a failure to meet basic needs is due to external circumstances out of their control.[4] With this in mind, we may replace the second criterion in the tripartite analysis with this alternative: *(2) in which their basic needs are reasonably expected to be met (exceptions being justified only when the expected failure to meet a basic need is due to external circumstances beyond the parents' control).*

At this point it will be helpful to consider the content of children's basic needs or essential interests. Many commentators maintain that what parents owe their children extends beyond a life worth living, suggesting at least partial lists of basic needs. Glover, for example, states that we owe our children a decent chance at a good life, which requires food and shelter, protection and kindness, stimulation, and encouragement of their personal growth and autonomy.[5] Bonnie Steinbock argues that we owe our children a reasonable prospect of being able to experience pleasure, learn, and have relationships with others—as well as good parenting, which involves being able to love and care properly for one's children.[6] Laura Purdy maintains that one should have children only if one can ensure that they will have a decent life with clean water, nutritious food, safe shelter, education, and medical care.[7] Note that a great many prospective parents in developing countries would be unable to meet this standard. By contrast with Purdy's concreteness, David Velleman proposes what he calls a "personhood-respecting standard": a provision for the child that expresses due appreciation for the importance of human life.[8]

We might, in the general spirit of these proposals, construct a tentative list of children's essential interests or basic needs. Although any such list will be somewhat vague and arbitrary, a sensible list will serve our purposes far better than no list at all. With this in mind, I suggest that children's basic needs or essential interests encompass the following: *nutritious food, clean water, safe shelter, protective clothing, and competent medical care when medical attention is needed; freedom from slavery, other forms of wrongful coercion, and physical abuse; education and adequate stimulation; opportunities to play and experience enjoyment; the opportunity to develop independent interests and gradually find their own path* (see Chapter 4's discussion of the right to an open future); *and the love, kindness, and attention of at least one committed, reasonably competent parent.*

Suppose we agree that this list approximately captures a norm relevant to parenting, one far more demanding than a worthwhile life but less perfectionistic than the very best an advantaged parent can provide. As suggested by the competing tripartite standards articulated earlier—which vary according to their different formulations of the second criterion—there remains a question about how we should conceptualize the relevant norm. Does it demand only that parents who are capable of providing for their children's essential interests do so? That would imply that parents who cannot meet some of these needs are off the hook. More reasonably, this approach would let these parents off the hook in those circumstances in which their inability to meet a basic need is a consequence of external circumstances and not their own character deficits or pathology. A far more stringent interpretation of the relevant norm, meanwhile, would be that individuals should not procreate unless they can meet all of these needs of children. So a prospective parent whose child would be unlikely to have reliable access to medical care should not procreate. This would mean that most adults in some developing countries who would be loving, attentive, and resourceful parents should refrain from having children. There is an acute tension between adequately protecting children by insisting that their basic needs be met and adequately respecting the procreative freedom of disadvantaged people.

The tripartite analysis that includes the final formulation of the second criterion seems to me far more reasonable. It insists that parents do the best they can with respect to basic needs, which seems appropriately demanding of parents and protective of children, while tolerating failure to meet basic needs where the parents cannot meet them due to external circumstances beyond their control, a concession to procreative freedom that is respectful of disadvantaged persons around the world.

But this tripartite standard still seems not quite right. For it seems to me that there is a basic need that should be non-negotiable: the love, kindness, and attention of at least one committed, reasonably competent parent. No one who is psychologically incapable of loving and being kind to their children should become a parent. The same goes for parents who, whether due to their psychological constitutions or competing commitments, are incapable of giving their child a decent amount of attention. And if a prospective parent isn't even reasonably competent to do the job of parenting, and does not have a partner to fill this roll, then he or she should remain childless.

Moreover, although some exceptions to meeting basic needs are to be tolerated, there must be some limit to tolerable exceptions. Imagine a couple who could offer love, kindness, attention, and competent parenting to any children they had, but found themselves in extremely poor circumstances. Through no fault of their own, let us suppose, their children would be slaves who were regularly subject to physical abuse and coercion, and who not only lacked access to appropriate medical care and education, but also would be deprived of nutritious food and clean water. The prospect of such extensive deprivation seems to make having a child in these circumstances a morally indefensible choice. Yes, there can be some exceptions to the meeting of basic needs, but not too many exceptions, as there would be in this case. On the other hand, the deprivations featured in this case make it hard to believe that the child's life could be expected to be worth living. Thus, I will assume that the idea that there are limits to tolerable exceptions to the meeting of basic needs is captured by the first criterion, that the child's life is expected to be worth living.

We will find in the next section that there may be good reason to modify our tripartite standard further by adding an item to the list of essential interests.

SAME-INDIVIDUAL CHOICES: WHERE PROCREATIVE FREEDOM CAN BE OUTWEIGHED IN FAMILIAR MORAL TERMS

In facing same-individual choices, a couple or a mother can either have a child with some significant disadvantage or have the same child without the disadvantage. Suppose a pregnant woman learns that she has listeriosis, a food-borne infection. Her doctor informs her that early treatment with antibiotics is effective, that she faces significant health risks if the condition goes untreated, and that the infection can cause miscarriage or premature birth. She and her partner understand this information and obtain a prescription, but for no particularly good reason they never get around to filling it. One consequence of their omission is the premature birth of their son, who has various associated health problems.

The couple's negligence is seriously wrong. Even if the child's life is worth living, the parents were in a position to give him a life without the health problems caused by untreated listeriosis and premature birth. He has been harmed by their negligence. Because there is both an identifiable *victim*—the boy who was born prematurely—and a clear instance of *harm*—his being made worse off than he would have been in the absence of negligence—the wrongness of the parent's choice is easily explained. Same-individual choices have this character of featuring an identifiable victim and a clear harm. Lacking at least one of these features, different-number and same-number choices pose greater challenges to moral analysis.

It is worth emphasizing that same-individual choices can concern a child's life circumstances rather than a medical condition. Imagine a couple who decide to have and raise a child in a beautiful but very remote location where no schools are accessible, and they do not provide homeschooling. More outrageously, another couple decides to have and sell a child into slavery. Even if the lives of the children in these and similar cases are worth living, the parental decisions are morally outrageous in a way that is easily explained: The parents either subject their children to substantial, avoidable harm (such as slavery) or deprive them of a benefit to which they are entitled (such as education). In both cases there is a failure to meet a basic need they could have met.

Let us revisit the tripartite standard defended in the previous section in light of judgments about these cases. The standard states that parents owe their children (1) worthwhile lives (2) in which their basic needs are reasonably expected to be met (exceptions being justified only when the expected failure to meet a basic need is due to external circumstances beyond the parents' control) and (3) doing more for them where the parents can without undue sacrifice. How can we capture the moral failure of the couple who negligently fail to fill a prescription, thereby allowing their child to be born prematurely with predictable health problems? Here there is a failure to provide adequate medical care insofar as the child in utero, whom the parents intended to bring to term, needed medical care no less than the mother did. Let us turn now to a type of case that proves harder to evaluate.

DIFFERENT-NUMBER CHOICES: WHERE PROCREATIVE FREEDOM CARRIES MORE WEIGHT

In a second category of procreative choice, prospective parents must decide between having a child with disadvantage and not having a child. The parents considered in the previous section all had the option of having the very child they did have, without the disadvantage in question: health problems associated with premature birth, lack of basic education, or life as a slave. By contrast, the prospective parents considered here must avoid having a child in order to avoid having a disadvantaged child because any child they could have would bear the disadvantage in question. Thus, restraint comes at what may be a very high price for the parents. Procreative freedom is much more at stake in different-number than in same-individual choices.

But just how much procreative freedom is at stake in different-number choices depends on details. So far, in speaking of the option of "not having a child," we have tolerated some ambiguity. The phrase can mean "not having any child at all, even by adoption." Or it can mean "not having a child who is biologically one's own," which is compatible with adoption. But even the notion of having a child who is biologically one's one admits of an important distinction: having a child who is *genetically* one's own—the child inheriting the genetic contribution of at least one legal or social parent—and having a child who is *gestationally* the mother's own in the sense that she carries the child in utero.

Consider some examples to illustrate these different senses of "not having a child." An African-American slave couple living in Virginia long before the Civil War, a couple from the "untouchable" class in India, and a black couple living under South African apartheid before there was any hope of abolishing that system—all faced a choice between having a child with a terrible circumstantial disadvantage or not having a child. There was no realistic chance of having a child who would be free of slavery, caste-based oppression, or apartheid; nor was adopting a child without the disadvantage possible. By contrast, parents who know that any child who inherits their genes will have, or face an unacceptably high risk of having, a terrible disease may decide that they must not have a child who is genetically their own. But they could either adopt an already-born child or have a child with donor gametes.

In assessing the importance of procreative freedom in different-number choices, how much moral weight should be given to the nearly universal, typically very intense preference to bear a child who is genetically one's own rather than adopting a child who is not? Adoption is possible in many cases where any new child a couple could bring into the world would face substantial disadvantage. But adoption is also an option in connection with more ordinary decisions about childbearing, at least among relatively affluent parents in developed countries: Parents could choose to adopt an existing child rather than bring a new child into the world. Indeed, for one who accepts a direct form of utilitarianism—according to which we should always act in the way that has the highest expected utility—it may seem that prospective parents should always, or nearly always, choose to adopt where they can, considering the vast unmet need among parentless children. I have some sympathy for the view that prospective parents have an obligation to adopt, if they can, before having a child who is biologically their own. But, at the end of the argumentative day, I accept neither any direct form of utilitarianism nor the strong thesis about obligatory adoption. Arguably, one reason to reject such an ethical theory is that it will invariably accord too little weight to procreative freedom.[9]

The value of procreative freedom, in my view, justifies many ordinary acts of procreation. This is true, I suggest, even where adoption is possible. When couples may choose between procreation and adoption, the latter is typically the more noble and generous choice. Where a couple could bring into the world a child whose basic needs would be met and who is likely to be free of serious disability, yet choose to adopt an existing child and provide well for her, they make a great contribution to humanity. But it is understandable for parents to prefer to bear their own child. Genetic narcissism, the desire to pass on one's own genes, is a significant psychological force that presumably arose because hominids who cared deeply about having their own offspring reproduced more than hominids who did not; and this biologically rooted preference is reinforced by culture insofar as heterosexual couples of childbearing age are strongly encouraged to bear children. Although not particularly rational, this preference is deeply human and hard to eliminate with rational reflection. Another reason to respect it concerns a distinctively female perspective. For some women, the experience of *pregnancy and childbirth*—as part of the process leading to motherhood—are central to their life plans. To adopt a child would permit the experience of motherhood, but not those of pregnancy and childbirth.[10] Thus, while adoption may be the more noble option where prospective parents have a choice, there are respectable reasons for preferring to procreate. The value of procreative freedom, I suggest, justifies honoring this preference in ordinary cases.

Matters are more complicated where procreation comes with the guarantee or high likelihood of serious disadvantage. In these cases, one faces a choice between bringing into existence a new child with disadvantage or adopting an existing child who needs a decent life. Suppose parents know that any child they bear will be blind. They can reasonably expect to meet the basic needs of their blind child, let us assume, but they also know that he is likely to encounter great obstacles in being unable to navigate the world visually. As argued in Chapter 4, it could turn out that a blind person will fare just as well as the average sighted person or fare just as well as she would have if she herself were sighted, but the odds are against these congenial possibilities. Meanwhile, the parents could meet all the basic needs of another child, who already exists and whom they could adopt. Adopting him would not create a new individual who faces the significant challenges of blindness. There is a case for saying, at least presumptively, that the parents should not bear a child they know would be blind when they can adopt a child instead.

On the other hand, there is also a case for judging it permissible to procreate in this situation. After all, as just argued, parents are not generally under an obligation to adopt whenever they can. It was also argued that parents who, due to external circumstances out of their control, would be unable to meet some of the basic needs of any child they bore could responsibly procreate so long as they could offer a worthwhile life and did the best they could in meeting basic needs. One might argue that it is more consistent with the tenor of those judgments to hold that it would be permissible to have a blind child, rather than adopt, so long as the conditions of the tripartite standard were met. With strong arguments on both sides, it is clearly a hard case.

At this point, one might call for an addition to the list of basic needs. Perhaps *freedom from significant, avoidable disability* is itself a basic need. If so, then the couple who elect to have a blind child rather than adopt would fail to meet this need. If they can adopt a child who has no major disability, then to create a new child with such a disadvantage would be, in effect, to produce an avoidable disability. Even if they adopt a child who has a major disability, they would meet her basic need for freedom from avoidable disability: The child already existed with the disability, which was in that sense unavoidable. Those who, in contrast to this reasoning, think that prospective parents who have the options of bearing a blind child or adopting may permissibly take the former course would decline to add "freedom from significant, avoidable disability" to the list of basic needs.[11]

Some parents face a different sort of dilemma: either bear a child with a substantial disadvantage or, adoption being unavailable to them, not have any child. Think of married slaves in the American South who know that any child they have will be born in slavery and likely remain in slavery her whole life. They cannot adopt a free child. If they can adopt a slave child, doing so would be better than producing a new child to share that fate, but let us assume this option, too, is unavailable. It would be most noble for the slave couple to abstain from bearing children rather than condemning a new child to a life of slavery. But, assuming they cannot adopt, the importance of procreative liberty would on my view justify their bearing a child—assuming it is reasonable to believe that her life would not be so bad as not to be worth living and that any failure to meet their child's basic needs would be due to external circumstances beyond their control. Freedom from slavery, of course, would be a basic need they *cannot* meet.

By now, it is apparent that there are some cases in which any child of prospective parents would face a major disadvantage, even if adoption is available and chosen. This is true in many cases involving slavery. It is also true with very elderly parents: Adopting a child won't make them any younger, so if there is any significant disadvantage to having very elderly parents, any child these parents have will encounter it. A similar point applies to prospective parents who are very poor and unlikely to escape poverty. We will return to cases involving elderly parents and poverty towards the end of the chapter. Let us turn now to a type of case that generates a special conceptual puzzle.

SAME-NUMBER (BUT DIFFERENT-INDIVIDUAL) CASES: THE NONIDENTITY PROBLEM

Introducing the Problem

Consider three hypothetical cases.

Preconception: A physician informs his patient and her husband that they should delay attempts to conceive because the woman has a medical condition that would likely cause any child she has to be moderately mentally retarded. If she takes a safe medication for a month, she can later get pregnant and give birth to a healthy child. Because she and her husband do not take this advice, they achieve pregnancy two weeks later, leading to the birth of a moderately retarded child.[12]

Prenatal: A physician informs his pregnant patient and her husband that she has a medical condition that, if untreated, will likely cause her child, if brought to term, to be moderately mentally retarded. The treatment he recommends, a medication, is safe and effective. The couple fully intend to carry the fetus to term, so they face a same-individual choice: The mother will bear the same child whether or not she takes the medication. Because the couple do not follow the physician's advice, the woman gives birth to a moderately retarded child.

Neonatal: A doctor informs two parents that their newborn has a condition that, left untreated, will probably cause moderate mental retardation. The doctor prescribes a safe medicine that can effectively treat the child's condition. Because the parents do not fill the prescription, the infant's condition causes moderate mental retardation.

Common intuitive responses to Preconception include the claim that the parents act wrongly and, more specifically, that they *wrong their child* by not preventing the disability when they could have done so with negligible cost to themselves. Another common intuitive response is that Prenatal and Neonatal are relevantly similar, morally, to Preconception. Derek Parfit termed this judgment of relevant similarity the *no-difference view*.[13] But attention to numerical identity reveals that Preconception is importantly different from Neonatal in a manner that makes it difficult to justify certain judgments of common morality, including the contention that the child in Preconception is wronged. (Preconception differs from Prenatal in the same way—if the biological view of our identity, defended in Chapter 2, is correct and assuming the woman is at least two weeks pregnant. To avoid controversy about criteria of identity, complexity about the exact time of our origins on a biological view of identity, and qualifications about the stage of pregnancy, I will exploit the more straightforward contrast between Preconception and Neonatal.)

The parents' negligence in Neonatal is an obvious case of wrongful child neglect. Had the parents provided their newborn a safe medicine, he would not have developed moderate mental retardation. If, years later, the child is able to reflect on his situation, he could justifiably claim that his parents harmed and wronged him with their neglect. But Preconception is different. On any contending theory of numerical identity (not just the biological view), had the parents delayed pregnancy, different gametes would have united in fertilization. Because of the necessity of origins—the fact that no one could have derived from a different pair of gametes than those from which she did derive—the result of the parents' delay would have been the birth of *another individual* than the child who was, in fact, born in Preconception. This child would seem, then, to be in no position to complain about his parents' irresponsibility, for he would never have come into being had they acted differently. Even one who doubts that coming into being can constitute a benefit should accept this point. For, certainly, coming into existence with a worthwhile life *cannot be worse* than never existing. It would therefore appear, at least at first glance, that the parents in Preconception act wrongly *but do not wrong their child*. How to make moral and conceptual sense of this is what Parfit called *the nonidentity problem*. This problem arises both in the context of reproductive decision making, as discussed in this section, and in the context of making decisions that affect future generations, the topic of Chapter 7.

The nonidentity problem creates a feeling of paradox in several ways. First, as already noted, many people believe that the parents wrong their child in Preconception. Some, no doubt, will abandon this belief upon recognizing that the child who is born is numerically distinct from the one who would have been born had the parents acted responsibly. Still, it is commonly assumed that wrongdoing requires a victim, someone who is wronged, yet this case apparently features wrongdoing without a victim. Second, the parents' behavior in Neonatal, in which the child is clearly wronged—since it is undeniable that the same individual would have existed had the parents acted rightly—seems no worse than the parents' conduct in Preconception. Now, if the child in Preconception really is wronged, contrary to what considerations of identity seem to suggest, that would dissolve the second puzzle: The parents' actions in Preconception and Neonatal would be equally wrong because the child would be (equally) wronged in the two cases. But, if, as Parfit maintains, the child is not wronged in Preconception, there remains the puzzle of why the parents' conduct in Neonatal, which has a victim, seems no worse. Further, if the child in Preconception isn't wronged, how can the parents' behavior be wrong? How can it be wrong to do something that doesn't wrong anyone?

In the context of reproductive decision making, the nonidentity problem threatens certainly widely accepted moral judgments. We tend to believe that it is wrong for prospective parents knowingly to bring into the world someone with a substantial disability when they could—without substantial costs to themselves or anyone else—bring into the world someone lacking the disability. Nearly everyone, including opponents of abortion (who would oppose aborting the fetus in Prenatal), would judge that the parents act wrongly in Preconception, where merely postponing efforts to conceive would allow them not to bear a substantially disabled child. By creating doubts about our intuitive reactions to Preconception and other cases, the nonidentity problem threatens to undermine common judgments about obligations to prevent avoidable disabilities.

In fact, the importance of the nonidentity problem extends much further. In response to reflections upon nonidentity in a variety of cases, Parfit argues that the part of morality concerned with benefiting and harming—or, more precisely, with the production of better and worse states of affairs (since the concepts of benefit and harm arguably do not apply in nonidentity cases)—needs radical overhaul. According to Parfit, we should understand this part of morality, which he calls *beneficence*, not in individual-affecting terms—not, that is, in terms of actions' effects on particular determinate individuals—but in the impersonal terms of how much good and evil (good and bad consequences) an action brings into the world. As we will observe in the following section, one strategy for addressing the nonidentity problem is simply to adopt Parfit's proposal regarding how to conceptualize beneficence.

Strategies for Addressing the Nonidentity Problem

In identifying and evaluating strategies for addressing the nonidentity problem, it may be helpful to highlight the claims that together create the sense that there is a problem that needs to be addressed. The key claims are the following:

1. *The precariousness of identity in relation to origins*: Our numerical identity is highly sensitive to our origins—such that, for example, you would not have existed had your parents delayed a couple of months before conceiving.

2. *The individual-affecting intuition*: An action is not wrong unless it wrongs at least one individual.

3. *The intuition of wrongful disability*: The parents' behavior in Preconception is wrong.

In drawing from the vast literature on the nonidentity problem, I will focus on those strategies that seem relatively promising. Several can be understood as rejecting one of the three judgments just listed. Because I regard the first of these, the precariousness of identity in relation to origins, as beyond reasonable doubt, I will not discuss strategies that deny this claim.[14]

Strategy A: Deny the intuition of wrongful disability (claim 3). The idea here is that, despite our intuition of wrongdoing, it is *not* morally wrong to have a child in the circumstances of Preconception. This strategy emphasizes the fact that the child's life, although characterized by a significant, avoidable disability, is worth living. It might explain the intuition of wrongdoing as resulting from an overgeneralization: We take the judgment that it is wrong to cause avoidable disabilities, which is generally correct where identity is maintained across the various options (as in Neonatal), and mistakenly extend the generalization to nonidentity cases.[15] Importantly, the present approach is motivated by the assumption that no other strategies for addressing the nonidentity problem succeed. If at least one does succeed, without abandoning the rather persistent intuition of wrongful disability, the successful strategy is to be preferred to the present one.

Strategy B: Appeal to harms caused to individuals other than the child.[16] It is often tacitly assumed in discussions of the nonidentity problem that any harms caused to individuals other than the child brought into existence, in cases like Preconception, are trivial. The present strategy reverses this assumption. Accordingly, one may argue that the parents' action in Preconception, which creates a child with special needs, may cause significant harms or burdens to other individuals such as the child's family, school, and broader society. If so, this could explain the intuition of wrongful disability—that what the parents do is wrong—without abandoning the individual-affecting intuition: that only actions that wrong someone can be wrong. This approach is driven by strong confidence in both the individual-affecting intuition and the judgment that a person cannot be harmed or wronged in being created.

I find this approach unsatisfying. First, it suggests that the wrongness of the parents' conduct in Preconception is contingent upon its being reasonably foreseeable that significant burdens will be imposed on others. If the parents openly accept any additional burdens, the costs to them would not seem to make their choice morally problematic. So the burdens that would be decisive would have costs to the broader society. Maybe these costs would be sufficient to explain the intuition of wrongful disability. But one disadvantage of the individual-affecting intuition combined with the judgment that one cannot be harmed or benefitted in being created is the implication that there are no wrongful life cases as these are usually understood—no cases, that is, in which an individual is wronged by being brought into being. In Chapter 5, such conditions as TSD and LNS were adduced in arguing that sometimes an individual is wronged by being brought into existence. Now, a proponent of the present strategy could modify it by allowing that a child is wronged when given a life that was predictably not worth living; this would leave the judgment that in cases like Preconception (in which the child's life is worth living), the procreative choice is wrong only to the extent that it harms individuals other than the child. While this move would increase the promise of the present strategy, I still find it hamstrung by an unnecessary attachment to the individual-affecting intuition. Moreover, the intuition of wrongful disability will be vindicated only in those cases in which some significant harm to other individuals occurs.

Strategy C: Claim that the procreative choice violates the child's rights.[17] This strategy, unlike the previous two, holds that, even though the created child is not harmed, she is wronged by the procreative choice. Specifically, it is claimed, her rights are violated. It is surely possible to violate someone's rights without harming her. Think of an easygoing student who is denied admission to a school dance because of her religious affiliation and later proves lucky in avoiding a catastrophic explosion at the dance. Due to her personality, she is not harmed by the rebuff; indeed, on the whole she benefits in avoiding the harmful explosion. Yet clearly her rights are violated. Another sort of example includes those innumerable cases in which a medical patient's autonomy is unjustifiably violated without any harmful consequence. So the present strategy is on strong ground in holding that one's rights can be violated even if one is not harmed.

On the other hand, it is on weak ground insofar as it is *in the interests* of a child in cases like Preconception—where life, despite the disability, is worth living—to have her rights violated in this way, suggesting that having the child in such a case does *not* wrong her. And exactly what right is violated by being brought into existence? A right not to be disabled? That possibility, plus the assumption that it is always wrong to violate a child's rights, would imply that every procreative choice in which a child will have a disability is wrong. But that is too strong a claim, as suggested by our earlier consideration of cases in which prospective parents cannot have any child unless they bear a child with a disability. One might claim that the relevant right is a right not to have an *avoidable* disability. But respecting that right would entail that the disabled child in Preconception who has a worthwhile life would never exist; another child would be brought into being. Again, it would not be in the disabled child's interest to have this right respected, so disrespecting it does not satisfactorily explain the intuition of wrongful handicap. This strategy seems inadequate.

Strategy D: Claim that the procreative choice harms the child in a noncomparative sense of "harm." All of the strategies considered thus far have accepted the assumption that a child created in nonidentity cases like Preconception is not harmed by being created. This assumption rests on a standard understanding of harm (see the discussion in Chapter 5), according to which one can be harmed only if one is made worse off than one was beforehand or would have been otherwise. Because the child in these cases did not exist prior to being created and could not have existed without the disability, the standard conception of harm implies that the child is not harmed by being caused to exist with a disability. The present strategy defends an alternative, noncomparative conception of harm that implies that the child is harmed in these cases.

According to a first approximation of this alternative conception, "[a]n action harms a person if the action causes pain, early death, bodily damage, or deformity to her. . . ."[18] On this view, a child who is brought into being with a disability is caused to have at least some of these harmful conditions and is therefore harmed. (The list could be plausibly expanded to include suffering and disability itself.) If this general idea is correct, then the procreative choice in Preconception negligently harms the child, explaining the wrong in nonidentity cases. As it stands, however, this conception of harm will prove inadequate in at least one class of cases: those in which an action causes someone to be in a bad or harmful condition, but does so by improving the condition of someone who was previously in a worse state. For example, a doctor causes a patient to experience moderate pain by giving him the best possible pain medication, which only partially ameliorates what had been severe pain. One way to improve this account of harm would be to state that the following is a sufficient condition of harming: One harms someone else if one causes her to be in pain, to suffer, to have deformity or disability, or to die prematurely *without improving a worse condition in that individual.*[19] (Since this formulation states only a sufficient condition for harming, one could allow that the standard, comparative conception of harm also states a sufficient condition.) The suggested modification would enable us to say that the child created in Preconception is harmed in being created while appealing to a rather plausible noncomparative conception of harm. Of the strategies we have considered thus far, this may be the strongest.

But, in my judgment, it does not solve the nonidentity problem. Even if we set aside any lingering doubts that the concept of harm makes room for the suggested noncomparative conception, this strategy seems subject to a problem that also thwarts the strategy of appealing to the child's rights. The problem is that appealing to a noncomparative conception of harm doesn't adequately explain the intuition of wrongful disability. Given that the child in question has a worthwhile life, and could not have existed without the disability imposed on her, she is in a position to be glad that she was "harmed" in this way. So it doesn't seem to *wrong this child* to bring her into being with a disability. Yet the procreative act seems wrong. So the latter intuition is not satisfactorily explained by appealing to the claim that the child was harmed. We still need an account of why the action is wrong.

Strategy E: Claim that the action harms or wrongs "the child" by widening the scope of the individual-affecting approach. Suppose we accept a standard, comparative conception of harm. It may seem to follow from this conception and the fact of nonidentity that the child in cases like Preconception is not harmed and not wronged. But perhaps this inference is hasty. One novel strategy is to argue that the procreative action in such cases harms or in some other way wrongs "the child" by broadening the scope of this referring term.[20] The idea is to exploit the fact that such descriptions as "the couple's child" can refer to different individuals in different possible scenarios involving a couple facing a particular procreative choice. The phrase refers to the child who is actually born, with a disability, in Preconception and it refers to the child who would have been born, without disability, had the couple followed the doctor's advice. Thus, we may say that the couple's actual procreative choice in Preconception makes "their child" worse off than the alternative of following the doctor's advice would have made "their child." In this way, they wrong "their child." This approach explains the intuition of wrongful disability in individual-affecting terms, construed broadly.

But does the appeal to the varying references of descriptive phrases like "the couple's child" really explain the wrong in nonidentity cases in individual-affecting terms? My sense is that it explains the wrong, if somewhat obscurely, while *abandoning* the individual-affecting intuition: the thought that an action can be wrong only if it wrongs some individual. The only individual falling under the term "the couple's child" who is affected by the couple's choice is their *actual* child. Yet this particular individual does not seem to have been wronged, for reasons already discussed. Rather than preserving the individual-affecting intuition, I suggest, this approach points in the direction of an adequate *non-individual-affecting* account of the intuition of wrongful disability. Before exploring this possibility, let us consider one more strategy that attempts to preserve both the individual-affecting intuition and that of wrongful disability.

Strategy F: Claim that the procreative choice wrongs the child by expressing inadequate regard for her.[21] Consider again the couple in Preconception, whose doctor advised the woman to take a medicine for two months before they attempted to conceive. For no good reason, they ignored this advice and conceived while it was still dangerous to do so. As a result, a disabled child is born. While the child has a life worth living, and cannot claim to have been made worse off by the couple's procreative choice, it is very clear that the parents did not make this choice *in order to benefit this very child.* Indeed, their conduct expressed a highly cavalier attitude about their procreative options and their likely consequences. In this way, the parents expressed a profound lack of regard for *their offspring—whoever it would be.* The present charge is lack of virtue, expressed through bad attitudes. Although the couple's disregard was not intentionally directed at the child they had, it was, in a sense, negligently directed at whatever child they might have. The child they did have, of course, falls under this description. In effect, the present strategy employs both the previous strategy (by focusing on any child the couple might have had) and the ethics of virtue.

This strategy seems to me partly successful. Unlike the previous strategy, which widens the scope of individual-affecting concern in referring to "their child," the present approach does not advance a dubious claim that their child was harmed. Rather, the charge is that the couple were culpably disrespectful of whatever child they might have—including the child they did have. Here, it seems, the child does have grounds for complaint: "My parents didn't give much of a damn about the welfare of their offspring—and that turned out to be me." Whereas the charge of harm may not stick to their actual child, the charge of insufficient regard does stick to him.

At the same time, this strategy seems insufficient to explain the intuition of wrongful disability. Although it explains an aspect of the parents' wrongful conduct—their disregard for their offspring—it omits something essential. Much of what seems wrong in Preconception is the fact that the parents negligently allowed an avoidable disability to come into the world. The disability was not avoidable *for the child who was born,* so he (unlike the child in Neonatal) was not a victim of avoidable disability, but the disability was avoidable in impersonal terms. The parents could have had, without any significant sacrifice, a child lacking the disability. There was something "harmful" about what they did, even if only in an impersonal sense given the fact of nonidentity. We therefore come to the odd notion of what might be called "victimless harm." While the present strategy partly explains the wrong committed in Preconception—and does so in individual-affecting terms—it doesn't capture the wrong of causing victimless harm.

Strategy G: Abandon the individual-affecting intuition (claim 2) and endorse simple consequentialism.[22] Simple consequentialism holds that the right act is that which has, or is expected to have, the best overall consequences. In doing so, it abandons the individual-affecting intuition and evaluates the consequences of our actions in impersonal terms. Simple consequentialism easily explains the intuition of wrongful disability by showing that the procreative choice taken in Preconception produces worse consequences than the alternative of following the doctor's advice and having a child free of disability. So straightforward is its proposed solution to the nonidentity problem that some may take its ability to supply this solution as a major argument in favor of simple consequentialism. And proponents of this approach consider jettisoning the individual-affecting intuition as involving no loss whatsoever. This intuition, in their view, simply overgeneralizes from the fact that everyday moral judgments of wrongdoing usually feature individuals who are wronged to the claim that all cases of wrongdoing must involve the wronging of someone.

Insofar as I agree that there is no rational basis for insisting that all wrong actions wrong someone, I find the strategy of embracing simple consequentialism, which so neatly addresses the nonidentity problem, more promising than most commentators seem to find it. At the same time, I believe it has too many problems to furnish a fully satisfying solution to the nonidentity problem. Notoriously, simple consequentialism—including its most celebrated version, act-utilitarianism—seems unable to account adequately for some of our considered moral judgments about human rights and the requirements of justice. These are problems regarding appropriate moral *constraints* on pursuing the best consequences. Simple consequentialism also has problems accounting for appropriate moral *prerogatives*. It seems, for example, excessively demanding of an agent's time and energy, judging her to have acted wrongly if she does any less than she could to make the world a better place—even if she does quite a lot. Of particular relevance to the present context, this approach does not seem to do justice to the value of procreative freedom. Anyone who is persuaded that these problems are fatal to simple consequentialism, yet is impressed by some of the strengths of consequentialism and feels no allegiance to the individual-affecting intuition, should be interested in the final two strategies to be discussed here.

Strategy H: Endorse rule consequentialism.[23] Rule consequentialism (RC) attempts to avoid key difficulties of simple consequentialism by revising the moral agent's job description. According to RC, an action is right if and only if it accords with a system of rules whose general acceptance by society would lead to the best overall consequences. The rules of this system are to be fashioned with a realistic appreciation of human limitations such as self-serving biases, a tendency to abuse powers of discretion, limited ability to estimate the consequences of particular choices, partiality towards certain people, and limited energy. With an eye on such human fallibility, the system of justified rules would include rules that accord with our understanding of rights and justice and rules that provide considerable personal space for developing our own interests and projects. Importantly, the protected personal space would include a reasonable measure of procreative freedom. With regard to the nonidentity problem, RC can take seriously the fact that people almost always think in individual-affecting, not impersonal, terms. It could therefore endorse some such rule as this: "When you plan to have a baby, make sure not to impose a disability on him or her if you can avoid doing so without great sacrifice to yourself or anyone else." The wrong in wrongful disability, as in Preconception, can be understood as a violation of this rule as people would generally understand it.

This strategy has considerable promise. But it inherits vulnerabilities associated with RC itself. Consider two ways of interpreting RC. On a standard, *foundationalist* interpretation, the rationale for RC is as follows: "If human beings were perfectly rational and could perfectly predict the consequences of their actions, then they should act in accordance with simple consequentialism, which, in principle, supplies the criterion of right action. Because, and only because, human beings have various cognitive and psychological limitations, it is best if they adopt RC, general compliance with which is the best hope for achieving the best consequences people are able to achieve." There are arguably two problems with RC, thus interpreted. First, when its proponents endorse particular rules, they hang their endorsement on the peg of an empirical assumption to the effect that, with human beings as we know them, general compliance with this rule will get us the best possible consequences. Such empirical assumptions are speculative and therefore uncertain. Second, the objections against simple consequentialism persist because RC, on this interpretation, takes simple consequentialism to be the ethical-theoretical foundation for RC. Thus, for RC, it really is conceivable that slavery could be justified in some circumstances, that it could be right to frame and execute an innocent person to prevent a bloody riot, and that it could be right to kill a healthy hospital patient in order to provide viable organs to several other patients in need. We "pretend" that these things could never be justified, according to RC (on the foundationalist interpretation), because real-world human beings will do worse in the long run if they feel open to considering such possibilities as moral. In response to this picture, the present objection is that these things are wrong not just in practice but also in principle.

Now consider an alternative, *pluralistic* interpretation of RC. On this interpretation, "Our confidence that slavery, judicial framing, and killing innocent patients for their organs are wrong need not depend solely on the belief that, in the long run, fallible human beings usher in better consequences if their rules prohibit such things. Rather, part of the justification for rules against these and other perceived injustices is that they are unjust (independently of consideration of consequences). That is, our considered moral judgments about rights and justice—as well as various prerogatives involving procreation and personal space more generally—provide some of the support for the rules fashioned in RC." Now, to afford our strongest moral intuitions a role in fashioning rules seems eminently reasonable: Doing so reduces pressure on the speculative empirical

assumptions made under the foundationalist interpretation of RC while quiet-
ing doubts about the moral adequacy of a purely consequentialist foundation.[24]
The only problem with RC on the pluralistic interpretation is that it might not
really be a type of consequentialism, since it abandons the thesis that, ultimately,
the *only* factor that determines moral rightness is conduciveness to the best consequences. RC, understood pluralistically, seems to be a hybrid moral theory
that mixes consideration of consequences with intuitions about justice, rights,
and personal prerogatives at its foundation. Thus, the theory might be better
characterized as "rule consequentialism-deontology." It is compatible with the
final strategy to be examined here.

*Strategy I: Adopt a hybrid view with both individual-affecting and impersonal
components.*[25] One who adopted simple consequentialism would construe all of
beneficence—all of that part of morality concerned with producing better rather
than worse states of affairs—in impersonal terms. Considering the difficulties
with simple consequentialism, as well as the unreasonable theoretical constraints
of a purely individual-affecting approach, an option worth considering is to construe beneficence in both impersonal and individual-affecting terms. More specifically, we might think of beneficence in individual-affecting terms when such
terms apply—namely, when our actions make particular individuals better or
worse off. But, in cases of nonidentity such as Preconception, we should think in
impersonal terms—that is, in terms of making the world better or worse than it
otherwise might be, depending on what actions we take. (At least, we should
think in impersonal terms when doing ethical theory; in practice, it may be best
for most people to think in terms of a rule that conflates impersonal and individual-affecting considerations, as formulated earlier in the discussion of RC.) Accordingly, in these cases, we can employ the aforementioned concept of *victimless
harm*: the bringing about of states of affairs that are worse than one could bring
about, even though no individual is made worse off. One need not assume that
all impersonal harming is wrong, as pure consequentialism seems required to
hold. What is wrong is causing impersonal harm when one can avoid doing so
without undue cost to oneself or anyone else, as in Preconception.

In a hybrid theory, what is the relationship between impersonal and individual-
affecting principles within beneficence or, more broadly, within a viable ethical
theory? This topic is too complex to tackle in any depth here. I will simply
advance a few remarks.

Both impersonal and individual-affecting principles count. In comparing
cases like Preconception and Neonatal, impersonal considerations in the
former and individual-affecting considerations in the latter have (at least
roughly) equal moral weight. In some other contexts, individual-affecting considerations may have much greater weight. For example, it is far worse to allow
someone who is enjoying a good life to die than to decline to bring into existence

someone who is likely to enjoy a good life.[26] As observed in connection with the asymmetry about reproductive decision making (in Chapter 5), the fact that a child one could bear would likely have a good life in no way obligates one to have a child.

One of the most intriguing features of the emerging theoretical picture is that impersonal and individual-affecting considerations are *nonadditive*.[27] When both apply, the individual-affecting considerations bear the full weight of the pair. That explains why the parents' behavior in Neonatal, which is individual-affecting but could also be assessed in impersonal terms (as we assess Preconception), is not far worse—perhaps not at all worse—than the parents' conduct in Preconception. If impersonal and individual-affecting considerations each retained the importance they carry in the absence of the other, Neonatal would be *far* worse than Preconception. But it is not. The individual-affecting principle kicks the impersonal principle off the moral scale when it is time to weigh in.

I find this strategy the most promising. It accounts for the intuition of wrongful disability as well as any consequentialist approach, but with lighter theoretical baggage—that is, without the problems associated with any purely consequentialist approach (whether simple or rule-based). It rightly treats the individual-affecting intuition as dispensable. By embracing both impersonal and individual-affecting principles, it acknowledges that both consequentialism and deontology (the general approach that understands right action at least partly in non-consequentialist terms) have important contributions to make to ethical theory without either cornering the market on moral insight.

Perhaps its greatest challenge is to persuade those who are initially skeptical that the broader ethical-theoretical picture can be completed, or even sketched, in a way that is sufficiently coherent, plausible, and reasonably free of ad hoc stipulations. A proponent of a non-hybrid approach such as simple consequentialism, RC on the foundationalist interpretation, or any theory that embraces the individual-affecting intuition might claim that the non-additivity of individual-affecting and impersonal considerations in the present approach hints that something is theoretically amiss. Such a thinker may harbor more general doubts about any ethical theory that doesn't have a unified foundation such as utility (consequences), respect for persons (or individuals), or the like. While I do not feel moved by either of the possible objections, others might.

Conclusion about the Nonidentity Problem

Having explored leading strategies for addressing the nonidentity problem, let us briefly take stock. First, the individual-affecting intuition, which states that *every* instance of wrongdoing must feature someone who is wronged, should be rejected. The very existence of nonidentity cases such as Preconception throws this intuition into doubt. It seems far more likely that the intuition has a grip on (some of) us because we grew up morally without thinking about nonidentity cases than because it is correct. Herculean efforts to preserve it may reflect an irrational prejudice against approaches to ethics that are even partly impersonal and consequentialist.

Relatedly, a genuine solution to the nonidentity problem will have to make a significant concession to consequentialism. The most promising approach, I submit, is the hybrid individual-affecting/impersonal approach. Perhaps RC, interpreted pluralistically—that is, rule consequentialism-deontology—provides the best theoretical background against which to develop a hybrid approach. At the same time, the attempt to explain the intuition of wrongful disability in terms of insufficient regard for one's offspring, an appeal to virtue, is also persuasive in at least some cases, including Preconception. While this strategy does not explain all of what is wrong in wrongful disability, since it cannot account for the wrongness of causing victimless harm, it does explain some of what is wrong in many cases—and in individual-affecting terms.

RECAPITULATION AND IMPLICATIONS

Taking Stock of Our Findings

In this chapter, we have examined the ethics of bearing and caring for children with disadvantage, focusing on cases in which the disadvantage in question— either a disability or a life circumstance—is substantial, but not so terrible as to make the child's life not worth living. Where a child's quality of life is expected to be so terrible, as discussed in Chapter 5, we have a *paradigm* instance of wrongful life: It is wrong knowingly or negligently to bear such a child, and to do so wrongs the child. In effect, the investigation of this chapter has sought criteria for a second category of wrongful life, which we can call cases of *wrongful disadvantage*.

In order to determine what constitutes wrongful disadvantage, we have had to consider what parents owe their children while bearing in mind different sorts of procreative choice. I argued that what parents owe their children can be understood in roughly these terms:

1. worthwhile lives
2. in which their basic needs are reasonably expected to be met (exceptions being justified only when the expected failure to meet a basic need is due to external circumstances beyond the parents' control); and
3. doing more for them where parents can without undue sacrifice.

As for the content of children's basic needs or essential interests, I suggested the following as an approximate list:

- nutritious food, clean water, safe shelter, protective clothing, and competent medical care when medical care is needed;
- freedom from slavery, other forms of wrongful coercion, and physical abuse;
- education and adequate stimulation;
- opportunities to play and experience enjoyment;
- the opportunity to develop independent interests and gradually find their own path; and
- the love, kindness, and attention of at least one committed, reasonably competent parent.

I suggested that the last item on this list was non-negotiable: If a prospective parent cannot meet this need and does not have a partner who can meet this need, he or she should refrain from becoming a parent.

A possible addition to this list—*freedom from avoidable disability*—was found to be debatable. Moreover, the phrase is ambiguous in a way that parallels the different kinds of procreative choice we considered.

In same-individual choices, the same child will exist regardless of what choice is taken. In these situations, procreative freedom is morally constrained by children's basic needs. In cases such as Neonatal, where parents blatantly fail to provide for their child's basic needs when they could have done so without any significant sacrifice, their wrongdoing is obvious. In Neonatal, we could invoke either the child's need for medical care or, more controversially, a basic need for freedom from avoidable disability as the locus of parental failure. The concept of avoidable disability applies unambiguously in same-individual choices.

In different-number choices, prospective parents will either have a child with disadvantage or they will not have a child at all. In these cases, procreative freedom carries greater weight than in same-individual or same-number choices. That is because a decision to override prospective parents' desire to have a child is likely to be more personally costly to them.

It was chiefly in view of what prospective parents often have at stake in different-number choices that I defended the more flexible understanding of parental obligations regarding basic needs. Rather than claim that parents must meet all of their children's basic needs or not have a child, I argued that they could be excused from meeting a basic need where (but only where) failure to do so was due to external circumstances beyond their control. Without this flexibility, we would have to judge that prospective parents who, through no fault of their own, could not meet the basic need for, say, medical care would be morally barred from procreating—a judgment that seems deficient in sympathy towards many disadvantaged people around the world. Another type of situation involves a couple or a single person whose only procreative options are to have a child with a major disability or have no child at all (unless they adopt). The value of procreative freedom leaves open whether this couple may responsibly have a child. If we believe that children have a basic need to be free of avoidable disability, we could judge either that (1) the parents *cannot* meet this basic need and are therefore off the hook of any expectation to do so, or (2) they can meet this need because the disability is *not avoidable* for their child. Again, procreative freedom carries more weight with different-number choices.

In same-number (but different-individual) choices, we encounter the puzzles connected with the nonidentity of the children the parents could have depending on how they decide. The leading puzzle was to explain why the parental negligence in Preconception is wrong, despite the apparent lack of any victim—and no less wrong than the negligence in Neonatal, in which there is clearly a victim. We found a satisfactory solution to the nonidentity problem. *The fact that we did so implies that same-number choices are morally comparable to same-individual choices.* So long as the disadvantage imposed by negligence is comparable in each instance, parents do no less wrong in same-number choices than they do in same-individual choices. They cannot justify their negligence by appealing to the fact of nonidentity. Nor can they cogently claim that the disability they imposed on their child was unavoidable. True, it was unavoidable *for that child*, who would not existed without the disability, but (unlike in different-number choices) there was no compelling reason to have *that* child rather than another who would have been free of disability.

"But wait," one might interject. "We left open whether freedom from avoidable disability was a basic need of children. Unless we decide that it is, on what grounds can we condemn the parents' negligence in same-number cases? It doesn't seem to violate any of the three conditions stated in the analysis of what parents owe their children." This is where an interesting observation can be made. Because the virtue-related wrong of insufficient regard for offspring is unable to account fully for the wrong in same-number cases, we must appeal to the idea of victimless harm. The wrong of causing victimless harm can be understood only in impersonal, consequentialist terms. It cannot be understood in individual-affecting terms. *That means that this kind of wrong, which characterizes nonidentity cases, cannot be explained in terms of what parents owe their children.* We are looking in the wrong place if we are looking at the list of parental obligations to their children. Ethics does not involve only what we owe each other: our children or anyone else. It also involves the impersonal project of making the world a better place.

Our investigation shows that there are two major kinds of wrongful life: paradigm cases, where life is expected not to be worth living, and wrongful disadvantage, where life is expected to be worth living but some other moral standard is breeched. Among cases of wrongful disadvantage, the wrong-doing of some can be understood in terms of parents' failing to live up to what they owe their children. In other cases of wrongful disadvantage, the wrong, or at least one aspect of it, can be understood only in the impersonal terms of failing to make things better when one could reasonably have been expected to do so.

Further Implications

Having established a framework for understanding the ethics of procreation, let us turn our attention to certain kinds of circumstance in which prospective parents may find themselves. This will help to add normative flesh to our skeletal framework. It will also enable us to address, however sketchily, some prominent issues in procreative ethics. Having given considerable attention to issues involving disabilities in earlier sections, here we will focus on life circumstances. With an eye toward contemporary relevance, we will further focus on circumstances that are realistic for prospective parents today—with one exception, to be discussed last.

VERY YOUNG PARENTS

Generally speaking, minors should not become parents. They are extremely unlikely to be competent in performing the duties of parenthood. And the demands of parenthood, assumed at such a young age, are likely to crowd out opportunities for education and the development of credentials and skills needed for secure employment. As a consequence, they and their children are very likely to bear the burdens of poverty. This is not to say that poverty itself is a reason not to have children, but that avoidable poverty—the result of poor family planning—is such a reason.

It is worth mentioning that my primary focus throughout this discussion is on family planning. In the case of very young parents, the idea is that it is unwise and irresponsible either (1) to attempt to become pregnant and have a child or (2) to risk becoming pregnant by engaging voluntarily in sex without appropriate birth control measures. I do not suggest that those who become pregnant, whether intentionally or accidentally, have an obligation to terminate their pregnancies. Whether they have such an obligation would depend at least partly on their beliefs about the morality of abortion. Those who sincerely believe that it would be unethical to have an abortion should not be forced or unduly pressured to do so. In the case of minors, however, their young age and presumptive immaturity may make it appropriate for close associates to engage them in a discussion of their options, the likely consequences of each, and even the moral arguments for and against abortion.

SINGLE PARENTS

Other things equal, it is better for children to have two parents who work well together in parenting than to have a single parent. But an enormous number of children are raised by single parents, many of whom do a great job of parenting. And many intact couples parent poorly. Although I lack empirical evidence beyond my own observations to support this contention, it seems that the difference between having one good parent and having two is considerably smaller than the difference between having no good parent and having one. What is really crucial is to have one loving, competent parent.

A hard question remains: Is it morally appropriate to *set out to be a single parent?* It is one thing to have a child with a partner and then become single. It is another to have a child with no partner in one's life or even in mind. Assuming that it is somewhat better, other things equal, to have two good parents than just one, one might argue that it is not acceptable deliberately to have a child alone. One ought to wait until one has a partner before having children, according to this line of thought. I disagree. Some people are in a good position to know that they are up to the rigors of parenting by themselves and do not have the luxury of waiting around for a good partnering relationship to happen. This is especially true where the prospective single parent is willing to adopt. Children waiting for adoption desperately need the love, attention, and support of at least one good parent; if a good prospective parent, though single, is available, he or she should be able to adopt. As discussed earlier, however, there are respectable reasons for strongly preferring not to adopt, so I am not prepared to judge that adoption is the only appropriate means to intentional single parenthood.

GAY OR LESBIAN PARENTS

There is no serious moral issue here. That is because there is no good reason to believe that homosexual parents cannot raise children as well as heterosexual parents. In the absence of any well-grounded objection to gay or lesbian parenthood based on children's interests, the importance of treating members of minority sexual orientations as fully equal citizens strengthens an already strong case for not discriminating against gays and lesbians who want to become parents. On a personal note, a college friend of mine, who is both gay and single, adopted a child at the age of 47. I am delighted for both father and son that they have each other.

ELDERLY PARENTS

There are two main sources of concern about relatively elderly people becoming parents. One is that they may not have the energy required for the exhausting demands of parenting young children. That may or may not be true, depending on the couple or single parent. The relevant criterion here is that a child brought into the world should have at least one loving, attentive, reasonably competent parent. Many elderly parents will pass this test. A second source of concern is that elderly parents, on average, have a shorter (remaining) life expectancy than younger parents. The worry is that children will be robbed of their parents at too young an age. But this worry should be put in perspective. A healthy American 60-year-old, for example, is likely to live twenty or more years. Thus, he or she is likely to be around long enough for their child to enter adulthood. This is the threshold I would recommend: If one is likely to live long enough to see one's child into adulthood, one should not be considered morally ineligible *on account of age* to seek to bear a child. It will be important, though, that the child have, throughout childhood, at least one parent who has the energy and ability to parent well. Thus, a 60-year-old who has no partner and has been diagnosed with a medical condition that will make him highly debilitated before any child of his would reach adulthood should not seek to bear a child (with a donated ovum and gestational surrogate) or adopt one.

POVERTY

As suggested earlier, poverty in no way excludes one from responsible parenthood. Those who are poor should not be excluded from the satisfactions of parenthood just on account of their economic status. The important thing for prospective parents of modest means, assuming that their children would likely have worthwhile lives, is to meet as many of their children's basic needs as they can (ideally, all of them). That means that if they face a genuine choice between conceiving now, when they cannot meet some of these basic needs, and conceiving later, when they can, they should postpone expanding their family if they can do so without excessive sacrifice. And, of course, they must be able to offer their children the love, kindness, and attention of at least one reasonably competent parent. But, in my experience, poor people are no less likely than wealthy people to be able to meet that non-negotiable need.

UNINVOLVED YUPPIE AND/OR NARCISSISTIC PARENTS

It is sometimes assumed that wealth is associated with a greater likelihood that parents will give their children good lives. It seems undeniable that wealth furnishes certain advantages for children that they might otherwise not have: private schooling or tutoring, skiing vacations, horseback riding lessons, nice clothes, and lots of presents, to name just a few. But there is no reason to believe that wealth is correlated with the virtues that enable one to be a loving, kind, attentive, and available parent. Indeed, great wealth is often accompanied by greed, the latter providing the motivation for the former, not to mention (for those who work for their wealth) a willingness to devote oneself single-mindedly and for very long hours to professional work. Imagine a couple, both of them corporate lawyers, who typically work from 9 a.m. to 9 p.m. and large chunks of weekends. Imagine that they decide to have children because "that's what people do at our age," intending to hire out most of the caretaking work. Suppose their greed is part of a broader pattern of self-absorption: They have trouble taking other people's interests and perspectives seriously. It is not unlikely that this couple would be incapable of meeting children's non-negotiable basic need to have the love, kindness, and attention of one committed and reasonably competent parent. If so, this couple should remain childless.

REPRODUCTIVE CLONING

My remarks on this much-discussed topic will be brief. Suppose, even if unrealistically, that reproductive cloning has become safe, legal, and affordable to many parents. Would it, or could it, be morally responsible for parents to use cloning to produce a baby? Doing so would involve extracting a somatic cell from one of their bodies, or perhaps that of a donor, introducing it into an enucleated egg cell, implanting the now-nucleated egg into the woman's uterus, and allowing the pregnancy to proceed. Could it be responsible for a couple or a single person to have a baby through cloning?

In principle, yes, because it is certainly possible that the parent(s) would be able to fulfill the parental obligations stated in the three conditions. The devil is in the details, and the details of motivation are of paramount importance. Some possible motivations for cloning are more compatible with good parenting than others are. So let us consider examples.

A couple wants to clone because they want a baby who is just like the father or the mother. Setting aside their failure to appreciate the role of environment in shaping the sorts of people we become, there are grounds for suspecting that this couple would not be good enough parents. For children's basic needs include opportunities to develop independent interests and gradually find their own paths, a point that is captured in the phrase "a right to an open future." Parents who want a child who is just like one of them, at least if they are prepared to steer the child's development accordingly should the child diverge from the cloned parent's mold, are unlikely to respect the child's right to be himself. Moreover, the parent to be cloned might be too narcissistic to parent well, which is hardly a plus even if the other parent does not have this limitation. Such parents should not have a child through cloning.

Another couple wants to clone a child, using a preserved somatic cell extracted from a now-deceased child, in order to replicate the child they lost. These parents, too, are at significant risk of not respecting their new child's right to be herself. If they are prepared to impose the image of the first child on their new child, they should not proceed with their plan. (The same may be said of parents who plan to procreate naturally, rather than by cloning, but are equally unlikely to respect a child's right to find her own path.)

A third couple wants to clone a child from one of their somatic cells not because they want a replica of the parent to be cloned or because they want to replicate some other person. Rather, this couple is aware that the parent in question is exceptionally healthy by genetic constitution—whereas the other parent has average health—and they would like their child to have the advantages of the same, health-conducing genome. This motivation is quite compatible with good parenting.

A fourth couple would like to clone because (1) their genomes, in combination, pose great risk of contracting a terrible disease or disability, and (2) they would like their child to have some genetic connection to them—that is, to one of them—without introducing, through donor gametes, the genetic material of someone outside the couple. Assuming this couple's genetic narcissism is not associated with a more global narcissism that would translate into inadequate love and attention for their child, their motivation for cloning is compatible with good parenting. Moreover, their desire to avoid imposing a terrible, genetically-based condition on their child is admirable.

These four examples suggest that whether it would be responsible to undertake cloning as a means to parenting must be determined case by case. The bottom line is whether the prospective parents can satisfy the tripartite standard. Now, some may fault my brief analysis for making no mention of either the possibility of social harm to the child created through cloning or the costs to society of permitting this way of making babies. As to the possibility of social harm, I assume that it is relatively minimal and certainly manageable, a point I would make in connection with children of single or gay parents and children produced through in vitro fertilization—all of whom bear some risk of being teased by unenlightened peers and of feeling "different." As for possible costs to society, Chapter 3's response to parallel concerns regarding genetic enhancement should assure us that such concerns do not constitute a persuasive case that it would be irresponsible for a society to permit reproductive cloning. Besides, our present discussion assumed that reproductive cloning was already legal (rightly or wrongly), prompting the question of whether prospective parents could responsibly avail themselves of this option.

For the record, I will close by stating my opinion that reproductive cloning should never become legal—and for a very simple reason that I have never seen advanced in the literature on this topic. In order for it to be appropriate to legalize reproductive cloning, a society would have to ensure that it is sufficiently safe to make the attempt on human embryos. In order for it to be sufficiently safe to make that attempt, a massive amount of animal experimentation—far more than has already been done—would need to be conducted. In my judgment, while reproductive cloning would expand the procreative options of human beings and could serve some respectable purposes (as suggested by two of our examples), the advantages it could offer are not so great as to justify the massive amount of harm to animals that would accompany the endeavor of making cloning sufficiently safe. Many animals in cloning experiments, probably the majority of them, perish before achieving sentience. But many die late in pregnancy, when they are probably sentient, and many die after birth, when they are surely sentient. Even those animals, produced through cloning who live for years commonly endure health problems and deformities that lower their quality of life. In my view, we should not impose such harm on animals in order to clear the path for reproductive cloning in human beings.[28]

NOTES

1. My nomenclature for the three types of choices follows Derek Parfit, *Reasons and Persons* (Oxford: Clarendon, 1984), pp. 355–57, except that I substitute "individual" for "person." Fetuses and newborns are not yet persons on the usage adopted in this book. Also, the same sorts of choices can arise in the context of breeding animals.
2. Jonathan Glover, *Choosing Children* (Oxford: Clarendon, 2006), p. 57.
3. As in Chapter 5, in referring to TSD I have in mind the infantile form. Non-infantile TSD presents less severe symptoms but occurs very rarely in comparison with infantile TSD.
4. Why would it be any fairer to judge that a prospective parent should refrain from procreating and parenting if the expected failure to meet a basic need is based on *internal factors*, such as a compulsion to abuse children, that are out of his control? A proponent of the position considered here will insist that being unfit to raise children, even if the unfitness is not one's fault, is a morally compelling reason to disqualify someone from parenting.
5. Glover, *Choosing Children*, p. 51.
6. Bonnie Steinbock, "Wrongful Life and Procreative Decisions," in Melinda Roberts and David Wasserman (eds.), *Harming Future Persons* (Dordrecht, Netherlands: Springer, 2009), p. 163.
7. Laura Purdy, "Loving Future People," in Joan Callahan (ed.), *Reproduction, Ethics, and the Law* (Bloomington, IN: Indiana University Press, 1995).
8. David Velleman, "Persons in Prospect," *Philosophy and Public Affairs* 36 (2008): 221–88.
9. This claim is advanced in Tim Mulgan, *Future People* (Oxford: Clarendon, 2006), chap. 1.

10. Thanks to Peter Caws for suggesting this point to me. Of course, a woman could intend to have the experience of pregnancy and childbirth with no intention of raising a child, for a woman could plan to procreate just for the sake of procreating and then give the child up for adoption. I take it that proceeding with such a plan would be thoroughly irresponsible—unless, that is, the gestational mother made arrangements with another individual or couple to relinquish the child at the time of birth and the intended social parents could satisfy the tripartite standard.

11. Or perhaps they would accept this addition to the list of basic needs but judge that in the cases in question, in which the child could not have been born without the disability, the latter was *not* avoidable. Hereafter, I will ignore this conceptual possibility.

12. Pregnancy with rubella (German measles) is somewhat like this case. A woman who has rubella at any time during the first 20 or so weeks of pregnancy is at high risk of causing the child to be born with mental retardation. Other risks to the child include motor retardation, malformations of the heart and eyes, deafness, seizures, and bone disease. The three cases presented here are simplified in order to allow easy comparisons among them. A similar triad of cases is presented in Dan Brock, "The Nonidentity Problem and Genetic Harms—the Case of Wrongful Handicaps," *Bioethics* 9 (1995), p. 270.

13. Derek Parfit, *Reasons and Persons*, chap. 16. All other references to Parfit's ideas in the present discussion of the nonidentity problem will be to this chapter.

14. For excellent overviews of the nonidentity problem, see David Heyd, "The Intractability of the Nonidentity Problem," in Roberts and Wasserman, *Harming Future Persons*: 3–25 and Melinda Roberts, "The Nonidentity Problem," *Stanford Encyclopedia of Philosophy* (entry published July 21, 2009).

15. David Boonin, "How to Solve the Non-Identity Problem," *Public Affairs Quarterly* 22 (2008): 127–57.

16. See David Heyd, *Genethics* (Berkeley: University of California Press, 1992) and "The Intractability of the Nonidentity Problem."

17. See, e.g., James Woodward, "The Nonidentity Problem," *Ethics* 96 (1986): 804–31.

18. Elizabeth Harman, "Can We Harm and Benefit in Creating?" *Philosophical Perspectives* 18 (2004), p. 93.

19. Cf. Elizabeth Harman, "Harming as Causing Harm," in Roberts and Wasserman, *Harming Future Persons*, pp. 148–50.

20. See Caspar Hare, "Voices from Another World: Must We Respect the Interests of People Who Do Not, and Will Never, Exist?" *Ethics* 117 (2007): 498–523. Cf. Rahul Kumar, "Who Can Be Wronged?" *Philosophy and Public Affairs* 31 (2003): 99–118 and Jeffrey Reiman, "Being Fair to Future People: The Nonidentity Problem in the Original Position," *Philosophy and Public Affairs* 35 (2007): 69–89.

21. Cf. David Wasserman, "Harms to Future People and Procreative Intentions," in Roberts and Wasserman, *Harming Future Persons*: 265–85.

22. Parfit considers this strategy while also noting several objections to which it is vulnerable.

23. See Mulgan, *Future People*. Mulgan ultimately argues that RC is adequate not as a comprehensive moral theory, but as a theory covering a large portion of morality, including reproductive ethics (chap. 11).

24. As I interpret his theory, Brad Hooker takes a pluralistic approach to grounding RC insofar as he allows the moral importance of giving priority to the worst-off to play a role in justifying the ideal set of rules (*Ideal Code, Real World* [Oxford: Clarendon, 2000], chap. 2).

25. Varieties of this approach can be found in Brock, "The Nonidentity Problem and Genetic Harms"; Glover, *Choosing Children*, chap. 2; Jeff McMahan, "Wrongful Life: Paradoxes in the Morality of Causing People to Exist," in Jules Coleman and Christopher Morris (eds.), *Rational Commitment and Social Justice* (Cambridge: Cambridge University Press, 1998): 208–47; and my *Human Identity and Bioethics* (Cambridge: Cambridge University Press, 2005), pp. 268–79.

26. McMahan, "Wrongful Life," p. 244.

27. I owe this insight to McMahan (ibid, pp. 243–44).

28. I refer any readers who doubt that we should take animals so seriously to my *Taking Animals Seriously: Mental Life and Moral Status* (Cambridge: Cambridge University Press, 1996).

Obligations to Future Generations

GLOBAL CLIMATE CHANGE AND THE QUESTIONS TO BE ADDRESSED IN THIS CHAPTER

The term *global climate change* refers to a gradual yet significant change in weather patterns around the planet over a period of many years.[1] The term is typically used with an emphasis on greater extremes of weather, and the weather change that has received the most attention has been the gradual rise of average temperature in oceans and in the air near the earth's surface since the middle of the twentieth century. Hence the popular term *global warming*, which for practical purposes is nearly interchangeable with "global climate change." The latter term draws attention to the fact that the weather changes include, in addition to warming, such phenomena as greater rainfall and a higher frequency of extreme weather events such as cyclones and tornados—even some events that may seem inconsistent with the term "warming" such as especially harsh winter storms. Global climate change is a matter of great concern because its predicted effects, if current patterns continue, include greater total precipitation around the world (though some areas will experience extreme drought), rising sea levels (thus severe flooding), a variety of changes in regional vegetation and climates, decreased agricultural productivity, and more intense tropical storms. It is feared that these effects will together produce enormous harm to humankind— and other species—with more devastating consequences for poorer nations.

Assuming for the moment, as some skeptics deny, that global climate change is a reality, why is it occurring? The answer implicates the *greenhouse effect*, in which solar radiation is trapped inside the earth's atmosphere by greenhouse gases, heating the lower atmosphere and the earth's surface. Natural greenhouse gases include carbon dioxide, ozone, and water vapor; without the greenhouse effect, there would be no life on the planet. Of present concern are human activities that increase this effect by introducing additional carbon dioxide, nitrous oxide, methane, and other substances. Standard modes of transportation, animal husbandry, emissions from factories and power plants that burn fossil fuels, and deforestation are principal human contributions to an enhanced greenhouse effect.

While skeptics are said to deny global climate change, we must distinguish two questions. First, have weather patterns in recent decades in fact demonstrated a significant trend associated with the term "global climate change"? Since that question is a bit vague, it can be helpful to focus on warming and reformulate the question this way: Has the average temperature in recent decades demonstrated a significant upward trend—as opposed to insignificant variations up and down of the sort that can normally be expected? An alternative way of focusing the first question would be to ask whether in recent decades there has been a significant increase in the occurrence (number and/or intensity) of the sorts of severe weather events predicted by the thesis that global climate change is occurring. Second, if there is a significant trend involving global warming, or severe weather events, is the trend largely down to human activities or does it represent the sorts of changes that occur with longer-term, natural cycles in weather patterns? Skeptics either answer "no" to both questions or answer "yes" to the first but "no" to the second. According to one skeptical school of thought, if there is a significant trend but it is not due to human choices and activities, there is little motivation to address the trend by making different choices. This reasoning may be challenged, though, to the extent that making different choices can mitigate the harmful effects of climate change *whether or not it is not driven by human activities.*

In the United States, public debate persists about the reality of global climate change and whether human activity is driving it. At this point, however, the debate seems to be perpetuated mainly by representatives of industries with a stake in avoiding costly changes to curb greenhouse gas emissions, politicians with close ties to these industries, and some influential ideologues in the media. Among scientific experts, there is solid agreement that global climate change is real and driven by human activity. This pervasive agreement on the facts is reflected in the reports of the Intergovernmental Panel on Climate Change (IPPC), a report by the National Academy of Sciences, and in statements by such bodies as the American Meteorological Society, the American Geophysical Union, and the American Association for the Advancement of Science.[2] In 2010, the National Oceanic and Atmospheric Administration demonstrated that the 2000s were by far the warmest decade on record—as the 1980s and 1990s had been, in their turns—dispelling any reasonable doubt that the warming pattern was significant. Around the same time, Environmental Protection Agency (EPA) administrator Lisa Jackson rebutted petitions to revoke EPA's finding that "climate change is real, is occurring due to emissions of greenhouse gases from human activities, and threatens human health and the environment." The petitions, she stated, were based on "selectively edited, out-of-context data, and manufactured controversy."[3]

If the broad factual picture of global climate change is relatively clear, how to address the phenomenon is considerably less so. The overarching ethical issue is this: Given the great harm that is threatened if we do not stem the tide of climate change, what should we—governments and/or individuals—do? We can approach this question by reframing it as the issue of what we, who are now contributing to global warming, owe to future generations, who will inherit its harmful effects. This brings us to the central topic of this chapter.

In bearing children, we bring new human beings into the world. Collectively, the procreative acts of a given generation create a new generation. And, of course, the new generation will go on to create another generation, and so on and so forth for as long as the human species exists. In a somewhat loose sense, we may say that a given generation creates all future generations by creating the next generation and, with it, the possibility of later ones. Moreover, any given generation creates—or at least greatly affects—the conditions of the world that later generations will inherit and have to live with. With some grandiosity, we may say that everyone who procreates helps to create the future of humankind and its world.

As emphasized in Chapters 5 and 6, no one who is created—brought into existence—has a say in the matter. A new human being is thrown into a life featuring conditions and circumstances over which she has no control. If we consider new human beings of approximately the same age, we may make the same point of whole generations. Now, among the circumstances confronting new generations are many such as the state of the climate that will greatly affect their quality of life. Because our choices so greatly affect the quality of life for future generations, it may seem intuitively obvious that we have moral obligations concerning the ways in which we affect the world that we leave our descendants. As for the content of these obligations, some, presumably, would involve the avoidance of future harm whereas others would involve maintaining environmental and other resources on which human beings depend—and perhaps other things of great value.

A plausible list of such obligations to future generations might include the following:

- To be responsible stewards of the environment, keeping it reasonably clean and habitable—for example, avoiding disastrous climate change and lethal nuclear accidents—and preserving adequate natural resources such as trees, oil, and other energy sources for future use;
- To be responsible stewards of our gene pool (for example, taking appropriate precautions in pursuing inheritable genetic modifications);
- To avoid disastrous overpopulation;
- To protect important components of human culture (e.g., literature, music, historical sites) or the cultures of particular societies (e.g., valued monuments);
- To protect important technological resources such as medical knowledge and engineering capabilities;
- To keep national debts manageable;
- To protect valued nonhuman species such as elephants and polar bears from extinction; and
- To protect the human species from extinction by nuclear war, uncontrollable and lethal epidemics, destructive post-humans (see Chapter 3), or other threats.

It is not among the aims of this chapter to defend a particular list of obligations to future generations. Here the idea is to offer a fairly plausible statement of at least some of these obligations, if indeed we have any.

In doing so, I do not assume the correctness of any specific moral theory or theory of justice. But I do make some moral assumptions.

First, I assume, as I have throughout the book, that we have *obligations of nonmaleficence* (nonharm). It is pro tanto wrong to cause harm. Nonmaleficence is the basis of our obligations to future generations to avoid nuclear disasters, lethal epidemics, devastating overpopulation, and other instances of harm—if, that is, we have such obligations and the concept of harm can be legitimately applied in nonidentity cases, in which different choices would lead to the existence of different people.

Second, I assume that if we have obligations to future generations, some will concern stewardship of natural resources and some will concern stewardship of cultural and technological resources. How such obligations are to be grounded in particular moral principles or theories is a debatable matter.[4] Rather than pursue this theoretical issue here, I will proceed to the central issues to be addressed in this chapter.

Whatever general moral obligations we have, they apply most straightforwardly in our dealings with contemporaries. Difficult philosophical issues confront the thesis that we have obligations to those who will exist only in the future. While some may find it pretty obvious that we have such obligations, there remains both the challenge of explaining how this is possible and the issue of how stringent these obligations are. Other thinkers may sincerely doubt that we have obligations to future generations. Both groups have reason to pursue the issues addressed here.

Do we have obligations to future generations? Careful philosophical exploration of this topic—and, more broadly, of justice between generations—does not have a long historical pedigree.[5] The first clear articulation of the issue of obligations to future generations may have appeared in Henry Sidgwick's 1874 masterpiece, *The Methods of Ethics*, but Sidgwick made no attempt to resolve the issue.[6] John Rawls provided the first systematic account of intergenerational justice,[7] but his account, as we will see, proves deeply inadequate. More than any other thinker, Derek Parfit has advanced the discussion of obligations to future generations.[8] But his approach, too, faces serious challenges. In my view, Parfit's contribution is most notable for highlighting the nonidentity problem and for exposing various theoretical options and some of the challenges they face, not for furnishing the most adequate account of our obligations to future generations. There is work to do.

The discussion that follows will be organized into sections that address the following questions:

1. How should we understand the moral status of future persons? Do they have interests, significant moral status, and rights? Can we have obligations *to* them and not just *regarding* them?
2. Are our obligations to future generations a matter of justice?
3. Even if future persons have full moral status, and our obligations to them are a matter of justice, should their interests nevertheless be discounted (count less than ours) because of their temporal distance from us?
4. In view of nonidentity, how can we explain the wrong of irresponsible policy choices and individual decisions that leave a compromised world for future generations?

THE MORAL STATUS OF FUTURE INDIVIDUALS

Future generations consist of future individuals, by which I mean individuals who will exist *only* in the future and therefore do not exist now. Do future individuals have full moral status and the rights that come with it? Do they have any moral status at all? In order to have moral status, as we saw in Chapter 2, a being must have interests. So let us consider whether future individuals have interests.

It might seem obvious that they do not. Individuals who will exist only in the future do not exist now. As "non-existent things," one might argue, they are not really things at all, despite the appearance that a noun phrase refers to them. In order for something to have interests, it must exist—that is, there must really be something to have them. This, the argument continues, is not the case with future individuals, so they cannot have interests.[9]

It may seem obvious that future individuals do not exist, especially if we stress the present tense of the verb, for they certainly do not exist *now*. But there is another way to consider the matter, which allows for the possibility that, in a sense, future individuals do exist. Consider the four-dimensional perspective developed by Einstein and embraced by many physicists.[10] From this perspective, time is not fundamentally different in kind from the three dimensions of space that we ordinarily perceive. Rather, the four dimensions together constitute a web-like continuum of space-time. If we think in terms of this continuum, we may judge that future individuals *do* exist, even if not "now." They exist, but seem inaccessible to us (who perceive space and time as fundamentally different types of continua) because they exist in remote regions of space-time. From this perspective, the apparent nonexistence of future persons is an illusion caused by our limited perceptual faculties. Importantly, future individuals are not merely possible beings; they are actual and therefore real individuals, however inaccessible they may seem to us.[11] Once we appreciate that future individuals exist, the proponent of the four-dimensional perspective concludes, we can attribute interests and moral status to them.

So, if the four-dimensional perspective is correct, we may responsibly assert that future individuals exist and, as bearers of interests, have moral status. This would greatly strengthen the case for the thesis that we have moral obligations to future individuals and, collectively, to future generations. But, given the state of controversy among contemporary physicists, it would be risky and question begging—especially for an amateur like me—to assume that the four-dimensional perspective is correct. There are models of physics that challenge the thorough causal determinacy embraced by this perspective and/or challenge the idea that time is not fundamentally different from space (and the thesis that there are only four dimensions). Quantum mechanics and string theory provide ample resources for such challenges.[12] So, for the remainder of this discussion, I will grant for the sake of argument that future individuals do not exist. I will also grant that the universe may be causally indeterminate, meaning that what will happen in the future is not entirely determined by prior states of the universe and the laws of physics; for a given state of the universe or a region of the universe at some time, more than one future state is possible. If this is the case, then *who* will come into being is not determined prior to acts of procreation.

That means that the identities of future people are impossible to know in advance—not only in practice, in view of our limited knowledge, but also in principle due to there being (as yet) no fact of the matter as to who will come into being.

We have assumed that future persons do not exist. From this it follows that they do not have interests, moral status, or rights since there is really no "they" to have these things. It may seem to follow that we cannot have obligations to future individuals. But this does not follow. After all, even though we do not know who will exist in the future, we do know—or at least we responsibly assume—that there will be future people. Once they exist, they will have full moral status with associated rights. I hold, and will argue, that we can have obligations now to future people in view of the moral status they will have once they exist.[13]

Many find this dubious.[14] They assume that we cannot have obligations to any beings unless they *currently* have rights or moral status. (Since the argument is nearly always stated in terms of rights rather than moral status, I will follow suit.) In effect, these thinkers make two assumptions. First, they assume the correlativity of rights and obligations directed to particular individuals: *A (a moral agent) has an obligation to B (some individual) if and only if B has a right against A*. I accept this assumption.[15] But those who think that future people's nonexistence precludes our having obligations to them make a stronger, more specific assumption, which I will call *the temporally bound correlativity thesis*:

A *now* has an obligation to B if and only if B *now* has a right against A.

If this thesis is correct, then the nonexistence of future persons, which entails that they do not now have rights, does preclude our now having obligations to them. But the temporally bound correlativity thesis is not self-evidently correct. Indeed, I see no compelling reason to accept it.

When future people come into being, they will have moral status and associated rights. That, in my view, makes it possible for us to have obligations to future generations. Our obligations concerning stewardship of the environment and so on concern how our actions will affect future people's interests. Again, they will have rights—whatever rights all persons have—so their present nonexistence should not stand in the way of our having obligations to them. These remarks present only a sketch of an argument against the temporally-bound correlativity thesis, yet unless there is a strong argument in favor of that thesis, we have good reason to reject it.

The strongest argument of which I am aware for the temporally-bound correlativity thesis proceeds as follows:

We must assume this thesis in order to avoid the absurdity that logically follows from denying the thesis. So let's suppose the temporally-bound correlativity thesis is false and, accordingly, that we may now have obligations to individuals who will only exist and have rights in the future. Let's suppose, for example, that we have an obligation to prevent elephants, a highly valued species, from becoming extinct and that, in a few years, we violate this obligation by allowing their extinction. Shortly after this happens, someone is born who in time grows up sufficiently to feel bad that there are no longer any elephants. Resenting the people who negligently allowed their extinction, he claims that they violated his right to the preservation of valued species. But this is perfectly absurd because *one cannot have a right to some condition that is impossible to fulfill*. And, because this person came into being after elephants went extinct, and did not have any rights until he existed, it was impossible (setting aside fantasies of cloning preserved DNA) to honor his putative right to save that species. So he had no such right. A similar absurdity can be generated in any case in which an alleged obligation correlates with an alleged right that cannot be held contemporaneously with the obligation. Thus, we must accept the temporally-bound correlativity thesis.[16]

This argument founders on the assumption that one cannot have a right to some condition that is impossible to fulfill. Suppose an elderly woman gives her son $50,000 for one specific purpose: to help pay for his child's college education. Suppose that the gift is made before the son has any child. The son, it so happens, is imprudent and needlessly spends the entirety of the gift with the result that he is jobless, broke, and realistically incapable of attaining any employment that pays better than minimum wage. Now that the $50,000 is gone, he cannot replenish it; at best, he can pay his bills. The son and his partner have a daughter, soon after which he becomes a single parent. (The partner either bolted or died.) Years later, the daughter is accepted to a university and, knowing of the earlier gift from Gramma, claims that she, the daughter, had a right to the $50,000 and that her father violated this right.

The daughter's assertion is cogent. She had a right to that money. Yet, once she came into being, her father had already blown the money and was unable to replenish it. This implies that (1) she had a right to something she could not have, and (2) the corresponding obligation existed prior to the time that she had the right. The second implication is unproblematic if the temporally-bound correlativity thesis is false. But that thesis is motivated by the claim, advanced in the argument just presented, that one cannot have a right to conditions that are impossible to fulfill. The first implication asserts that one can have such a right. I suggest that one can—precisely in cases in which the right in question *could have been* honored through the correct choices. The man could and should have preserved the $50,000 for the child he would have. Squandering the funds violated his obligation. Her right, which did not exist until later when she came into being, was to a condition—the availability of that money—that was rightfully hers. It is irrelevant to her having the right whether she could, in fact, have had it fulfilled when it was time for college. What is relevant is that her father could have fulfilled his obligation and made the money available to her. This suggests that the earlier argument for the temporally-bound correlativity thesis is unsound.

For the remainder of the chapter, then, I will assume that the present nonexistence of future people poses no obstacle to our having obligations to them, considered either collectively or as individual rights-holders. That, of course, leaves open the possibility of other theoretical obstacles. But, as we will see, they pose challenges to the thesis that we have obligations to *particular individuals* existing in the future and/or to the thesis that whatever obligations we may have regarding future generations are obligations of primary importance that should carry full moral weight in our deliberations. They do not put in doubt the more modest, enormously commonsensical claim that we have obligations *regarding* future generations. And while the nonidentity problem may be understood as presenting an obstacle to the claim that we can have obligations *to* future generations (even considered as a collective), our discussion of the nonidentity problem in Chapter 6 sets us up to solve it in the context of future generations. Hereafter I assume that we have obligations *regarding* future generations and that these obligations are directed *to* future generations *at least as they are considered as a collective.*

IS WHAT SORT OF WORLD WE LEAVE FUTURE GENERATIONS A MATTER OF JUSTICE?

We have obligations regarding future generations to take appropriate care of the world that we leave them. But perhaps the relevant obligations are obligations to future generations *considered vaguely as a mass of humanity whom we ought to help, or at least not harm, if possible.* Perhaps we do not have obligations to future people *considered as individuals*, in which case their rights may not include rights *against us*. (The correlativity thesis we accepted earlier was that A has an obligation to B, a particular individual, if and only if B has a right against A.) The possibility that future persons do not have rights against us may, in view of the close conceptual connections between rights and justice, motivate doubts that our obligations regarding future generations are a matter of *justice*.

Moral philosophers as diverse in their theoretical orientations as Mill and Rawls have asserted that the moral demands of justice are especially urgent, and few of their contemporary colleagues would disagree.[17] If, therefore, our obligations to future generations are *not* a matter of justice—but are instead a matter of humanity (being humane)—perhaps these obligations have a secondary importance in comparison with the demands of justice. As Brian Barry states in considering this possibility, "Humanity requires that we respond to others' needs whereas justice requires that we give them their due. If something is due you, you do not have to show that you need it or that you will make better use of it than other possible claimants."[18] If our obligations to future generations are only a matter of humanity, then our justice-based obligations to currently existing individuals are more important. We *owe* our contemporaries whatever they are *due* in accordance with their *rights* as a matter of *justice*. By contrast, one might argue, we should make reasonable efforts to avoid harming future generations and to leave them decent natural and non-natural resources, but doing so is less important than fulfilling our justice-based obligations to contemporaries. Perhaps the rights that future people will possess will be exclusively rights against each other. If so, then we do not have obligations to future people as individual rights-holders. Rather, our obligations to future generations are directed to them considered as a collective, just as, one might plausibly argue, our obligations to assist the (presently existing) needy are directed to them considered as a collective rather than to particular needy individuals—who would then have rights against us.

How might this play out? Suppose that someone who believes that obligations to future generations are a matter of humanity, but not justice, embraces a vision of justice that supports a robust welfare state. This thinker might reason as follows: "If honoring present people's rights to adequate health care and education, decent wages or unemployment benefits, and social security is very taxing to a nation's economy, as seems likely, then our humanitarian obligations to leave a strong economy, a healthful climate, and so forth for future generations may have to be deemphasized. Justice for present people may require saddling future people with heavy debts and/or the effects of global climate change." From at least some ethical-theoretical perspectives, then, the stakes are high in addressing the question of whether our obligations to future generations are a matter of justice.

Are our obligations to future generations a matter of justice? Let us first consider reasons to think not before turning to considerations that tilt in the opposite argumentative direction.

The two major reasons to doubt that our obligations to future generations are based in justice are (1) a lack of reciprocity between generations of people who are not contemporaries (that is, they do not overlap at all in time) and (2) a great asymmetry in power. For it is commonly asserted that what Rawls called the "circumstances of justice"—the necessary conditions for relations of justice to obtain—include reciprocity and a rough balance of power among parties.[19] The lack of reciprocity involves the fact that two non-overlapping generations cannot cooperate with each other for the simple reason that when one generation exists, the other does not. Relatedly, if one generation does something that materially benefits another generation, it must always be the later generation that is the beneficiary; that generation cannot materially benefit the earlier one, which no longer exists.[20] In sum, there can be no give and take between two non-overlapping generations, hence no reciprocity. Meanwhile, the earlier of two such generations has great power over the later one, being able to influence the state of its environment, economy, and so on. Indeed, the earlier generation has considerable control over the very existence of later generations by influencing the *numbers* of people who come into being—in the extreme case of possible annihilation, *whether* they come into being at all—and, as explained more fully in connection with the nonidentity problem, the *identities* of who will come to be. By contrast, the later generation has no such power over the earlier one, being unable to affect it in comparable ways. In this sense, there is lacking the rough equality of power that is commonly regarded as a circumstance of justice. Characterized by neither reciprocity nor a balance of power, relations between non-overlapping generations cannot be relations of justice. Thus, the argument concludes, any obligations we may have to future generations are not a matter of justice.

This is a powerful argument, but I believe that several considerations should lead us to reject it. First, while the claim that relations of justice require reciprocity and a balance of power has a ring of plausibility, it is not self-evidently correct. Perhaps the ring of plausibility is sounded by the fact that reciprocity and balance of power characterize *paradigm* instances—that is, the standard and least controversial instances—rather than *all* instances, of relations of justice. It seems at least as plausible on its face to claim that *justice is involved whenever one party can substantially affect the most vital interests of another party who has full moral status and rights*. This is our situation in relation to future generations.

Moreover, several implications of the view that relations of justice require reciprocity and rough equality of power—call this *the classical view (of the circumstances of justice)*—are very difficult to believe. Before considering the implications, let us note that the classical view is at home in the social contract tradition in moral and political philosophy. This tradition, which traces back at least to early modern philosophy, has developed in many different directions while addressing a variety of issues including the basis and limits of governmental authority (Hobbes, Locke), the principles of justice at the level of basic societal institutions (Rawls), and the principles of moral conduct among persons (Scanlon).[21] Relevant to our discussion is the general idea that the demands of justice are represented by the terms that would be agreed upon in a hypothetical social contract. Importantly, the classical view stems from that part of the social contract tradition that construes the contract as an agreement constructed *on the basis of mutual advantage*.[22] The motivation for limiting one's own liberty (agreeing to obey the law and not to murder, steal, etc.) is that it is in one's interest to do so on the condition that other people agree to the same limits for themselves. Everyone benefits if everyone behaves. But here, crucially, "everyone" includes those who both motivated and permitted to go to the bargaining table in the first place: those and only those individuals (1) who have something to lose if others do not behave *and* (2) who pose a threat to others if they do not submit to the terms of a social contract. Hence the assumption that parties to any social contract are roughly equal in power. As Rawls puts it in characterizing those individuals who are to be imagined as contractors, they are "roughly similar in physical and mental powers; or at any rate, their capacities are comparable in that no one among them can dominate the rest."[23] This conception of justice implies that if members of group A are not powerful enough to force members of group B to the bargaining table—or, equivalently, to pose a threat that will earn them an invitation to the table—then there are no claims of justice on A's behalf against B.

This general implication of the classical view that justice is grounded entirely in mutual advantage is deeply problematic, as becomes evident when we consider several specific implications. Consider, first, the undeniable fact that European settlers in the Americas and the native population were not roughly equal in power. An implication of the classical view is that the subjugation of Native Americans by the settlers—involving quasi-genocide, the forcible appropriation of land on which the natives lived, innumerable instances of cruelty, and exploitation through misleading treaties—involved no injustice. A similar observation may be advanced regarding the American institution of slavery. Since whites held massively more power than the Africans they enslaved and dominated, it follows from the classical view that American slavery was not unjust. I suggest, on the contrary, that what European settlers did to Native Americans and, later, to African-American slaves provide rather clear instances of injustice despite the great disparity in power between the two parties in each case.[24]

Gross inequality in power also characterizes the relationship between individuals with severe mental or physical disabilities and individuals lacking such disabilities. Thus, the classical view implies that how society treats the severely disabled never involves an issue of justice. This implication is scarcely more credible than the implications regarding Native Americans and slaves.[25] Similar arguments can be advanced on behalf of weak nations in relation to super-powers, young children in relation to adults (unless children are protected by the terms of justice on the strength of their potential to become adults), and, more controversially, nonhuman animals in relation to human beings. It is not essential to the success of my argument that one find all such implications of the classical view unacceptable. It suffices to note that the doctrine has several thoroughly implausible implications. This places in doubt the thesis that relations of justice require reciprocity and a balance of power. If this thesis is incorrect, then it cannot support the claim that our obligations to future generations are beyond the concerns of justice.

In challenging the classical view of the circumstances of justice, I have traced its roots to the social contract tradition. But, as mentioned earlier, this tradition has developed in different directions; and not all contract theorists regard the social contract as grounded simply or primarily in mutual advantage. Indeed, one finds a departure from this view in Rawls himself. Despite his explicit endorsement of the classical view of the circumstances of justice, Rawls suggests a different, far more Kantian view in his conception of the "original position," in which contractors are imagined to formulate the principles of justice.[26] Contractors in the original position are imagined as not knowing their own social positions, wealth, talents, and other bias-inviting facts about themselves, so that the agreement they reach will be impartially acceptable and *fair*.[27] Thus, Rawls, who refers to his view as "justice as fairness," implies that justice (fairness) has a role in determining the conditions in which contractors may each pursue their self-interest through bargaining. This means both that justice is not simply a product of a hypothetical contract—is not entirely a social construction—and that justice cannot be entirely reduced to mutual advantage. This last point clears theoretical space for the inclusion under the terms and protections of justice individuals who are *not* roughly equal in power to the most typical contractors, or the majority of contractors, even if Rawls did not extend his theory in this direction. One who holds a more or less Rawlsian view of justice should reject the classical view of the circumstances of justice, in view of its implausible implications and dubious theoretical motivation, and move in the more Kantian direction just noted.

In contrast to Rawls, Scanlon takes his theory some distance in this direction, explicitly including, for example, severely mentally incapacitated individuals under the terms of the social contract.[28] Whether he would characterize our obligations to such individuals as a matter of justice—rather than simply a matter of moral right and wrong—is less clear. In any case, on Scanlon's view, an action is right if and only if it accords with principles that no one could reasonably reject. The central concern of this sort of contract theory is with moral agents' being able to justify their actions to each other. This creates an opening for the inclusion of future individuals among those who are protected by the social contract (enjoying the priority that the term "justice" conveys). For, as two commentators put it, "[w]hen deciding how to act, I can ask myself whether future people who are affected by my actions might reasonably reject a principle permitting those actions."[29]

Thus, we find that plausible extensions of what are probably the two most esteemed contract theories of the present era, those of Rawls and Scanlon, can accommodate the thesis that our obligations to future generations are a matter of justice. I make this point not because I assume that some version of contract theory is correct, but because this theoretical tradition is the source of the present argument for denying justice-based obligations to future generations. The thesis that obligations to future generations are a matter of justice is also supported by the claim, which we found at least as plausible on its face as the classical view of the circumstances of justice, that actions that substantially affect the most vital interests of individuals with full moral status are matters of justice. That we have justice-based obligations to future generations receives further support from the fact that the main ground for doubting it, the classical view, has extremely dubious implications such as the implication that European settlers' treatment of Native Americans and the Africans they enslaved involved no injustice. Together, these considerations undermine the claim that our obligations to future generations are not a matter of justice and are therefore of secondary moral importance. Knowing of no stronger argument for this claim, and assuming for now that the nonidentity problem admits a satisfactory resolution, I submit that we have justice-based obligations to future generations.

SHOULD THE WELL-BEING OF FUTURE PERSONS COUNT LESS THAN OURS?

Returning to the topic of global climate change will help to motivate our next issue. We contribute to climate change by using massive amounts of electricity, by driving gas-consuming vehicles with low fuel efficiency, and by purchasing products whose manufacture or transport consumes energy and/or directly releases greenhouse gases into the atmosphere. Among these products, meat may be the most costly to produce in terms of its contribution to climate change. We can reduce the damaging effects of climate change by driving less, insulating our homes, curtailing our use of electrical appliances, reducing meat consumption, and so on. At a policy level, we can take such measures as establishing fuel-efficiency standards for cars and energy-efficiency standards for light bulbs, measures that increase short-term costs. Such individual and policy choices entail sacrifices. How much are we obliged to sacrifice? That depends in part on how we much moral weight we should assign the interests of future persons.

This brings us to our question. Should we, in determining what we owe future generations, *discount* future goods—that is, count the goods of future individuals less than the goods of present individuals? A variety of grounds have been offered on behalf of the proposal for discounting future goods. Before we consider the more significant grounds, a distinction between two kinds of discounting is worth noting.[30] One kind is *pure discounting*: the assignment of less moral importance to the *interests*—collectively, the *well-being*—of future persons. This kind of discounting challenges the idea that everyone's interests ought to receive equal, impartial consideration. A second kind of discounting, often embraced by economists, is the discounting of *commodities* or the material goods and services that people consume. One can consistently discount commodities while embracing equal consideration and avoiding pure discounting. Here we will consider only pure discounting, which is the more central issue from the standpoint of ethics. (Also, I lack the competence in economics that is needed to address the discounting of commodities.)

In considering arguments for and against pure discounting, it is appropriate to begin with a presumption in favor of equal consideration for all. The basic idea of equal consideration—which assigns equal moral weight or importance to everyone's comparable interests—is a point of departure common to contemporary ethical theories. Consequentialism, for example, specifies the idea of equal consideration by assigning everyone's interests, well-being, or happiness equal weight in assessing the morality of particular actions in terms of their consequences. Deontological theories specify the idea of equal consideration in different terms such as equal rights, equal protection by moral principles, and the like. Virtue ethics, to the extent that it generates directives for action, makes similar assumptions even if in different terms. So the basic idea of equal consideration is not particularly controversial.

A presumption in favor of including future persons within the scope of equal consideration seems natural in view of the conclusion, reached earlier, that future persons will have full moral status. True, they do not *now* have full moral status because they do not *now* exist. But we have already seen that their futurity does not stand in the way of our having obligations to them, and we have found that these obligations are a matter of justice. These points cohere well with the idea that future persons should be presumed to fall under the scope of equal consideration—or, equivalently, that there is a presumption against pure discounting of their interests. But let us consider the arguments in favor of such discounting.

One argument appeals to democratic preferences. It is well-known on the basis of people's behavior, according to the argument, that most people care more about their present well-being than about their future well-being; and they certainly care more about their present and nearer-term well-being than they care about the well-being of people in the distant future. In view of this majority preference, which amounts to a discounting of future interests, the appropriate policy response would be to apply some sort of discount rate to the well-being of future persons. Not to do so would be undemocratic.

This argument, however popular it may be among economists, is obviously unsound. It conflates morally defensible policy choices with those responsive to majority preferences. Suppose the majority of Americans today wanted to force Native Americans to work in labor camps. Instituting this preference would violate rights and constitute an injustice, even if 99 percent of Americans preferred this course. (I am reminded of the perfectly absurd response given by the owner of the Washington Redskins football team when a complaint emerged that the team name was demeaning to Native Americans: A majority of Redskin fans, he stated, are not offended by the name and do not want it changed.) Democracy requires representative government, whose members are elected through voting, but democracy does not in general require instituting majority preferences—and cannot legitimately do so when they violate people's rights. Because the argument from democratic preferences takes into account only the preferences of living persons while ignoring the rights and interests of future persons, it is open to a charge of systematic injustice to the latter. As we have seen, our obligations to future generations are a matter of justice.

A distinct argument appeals to special relations. It is a tenet of common morality that we may appropriately favor, at least in some contexts, the interests of those with whom we have special relations. Parents, for example, typically and quite rightly favor their own children over other people's children. Friends may appropriately devote greater time and energy to helping friends than to helping strangers. Members of a particular community (e.g., local, national, religious) often stand in cooperative relations with each other and on this basis have special or stronger obligations to community members. Similarly, according to the argument, present people have closer emotional and social bonds to their contemporaries and those who will come into existence during their lifetimes; the more remote in time a future cohort is, the less closely we are related to it in relevant ways. This justifies a discount rate for future persons' well-being.

This is a more respectable argument than the appeal to democratic values. It is certainly correct that special relations often justify special treatment. Indeed, when special relations justify such partiality, there does not seem to be any incompatibility with a broad commitment to equal consideration. My prerogative to favor my daughter's interests over those of other children in no way implies that my daughter has higher moral status.

Crucially, the clear instances of justified, relationship-based preferential treatment seem to involve instances of *benefitting*.[31] Parents are entitled to support and help their children more than other children, but they may not *harm* other children any more than they may their own. Americans may have special reason to contribute to the welfare of other Americans—say, indirectly, through the use of their tax contributions—but they should not be more casual about harming people from other countries. This association of justified partiality with benefit is important because many of our obligations to future generations are obligations not to *harm* them, as discussed earlier.

Moreover, the asserted inverse correlation between relatedness in the relevant sense and the passage of time is loose. For example, I may justifiably feel more closely related to great great grandchildren I will never know than with currently existing individuals on other continents whom I will never meet and whose very languages I have never heard of. This suggests that a general time-based discount rate for the interests of future persons would be too crude an approach, if special relations justified pure discounting in the first place.

We turn now to what may be the two strongest arguments in favor of discounting the well-being of future persons. The first of these appeals to the prediction that, due to economic growth, future generations will be wealthier, materially better off, than we are. There is a virtual consensus among economists that this prediction is justified: Almost without exception, our economy grows every year and, over the longer term, economic growth is virtually guaranteed. If this is correct, then sacrifices that we make today for the benefit of future generations would involve the less wealthy sacrificing to promote the interests of the more wealthy, analogous to a regressive taxation scheme in which the poor are taxed in order to provide funds for the wealthy. In order to avoid a regressive approach to future generations, we should apply a discount rate of future well-being. This approach alone will permit us to be fair to ourselves.

In response to this argument, let us note first that it does not justify discounting people's well-being in the future just because it comes in the future; rather, it justifies such discounting because future people are expected to be materially better off than we are. In effect, this argument presupposes a *prioritarian* principle of justice: that it is pro tanto morally right to benefit those who are less well off rather than those who are better off. I believe there is much to be said in support of such a principle and grant its validity here. Nevertheless, for several reasons, I do not believe it justifies pure discounting.

First, the argument assumes that long-term patterns of economic growth will continue indefinitely. This might be doubted. For one thing, the Earth's resources—at least most of them—are not limitless. Although technological developments allow increasingly efficient use of limited resources, and some resources such as solar energy are effectively unlimited, it is an open question both how far technological breakthroughs can help us improve the productivity of limited resources and to what extent we will, in fact, take advantage of the effectively unlimited resources. At the time of this writing, there is some significant doubt about the long-term sustainability of our economic system and even more doubt about the sustainability of our environmental policies such as those that effect global climate change. So, the assumption that future generations will be wealthier than we are does not seem entirely safe. At the same time, I should note that some very good scholars think otherwise.[32] They assume that advances in technological capability will more than compensate for diminishing resources, effects of climate change, and increased population.

Even if it were a perfectly safe bet that future generations will be wealthier, it would not follow that they will be better off in the sense of enjoying greater well-being. In Chapter 4, I argued that human well-being could be understood in terms of (undeluded) life-satisfaction. I am not aware of any good evidence that later generations have greater life-satisfaction—are happier—than earlier generations. In fact, some evidence suggests that they are not.[33] I do not doubt that, within a given generation, those individuals whose basic needs are satisfied tend, on average, to be happier than those who have many unmet basic needs. But that does not suggest that a more prosperous later generation is on average happier—more precisely, enjoys greater (undeluded) life-satisfaction—than an earlier generation, in which case they are not better off in terms of well-being, the terms relevant to pure discounting.

Moreover, a prediction that future generations will be better off than earlier generations says nothing about how their large bounties will be *distributed*. Thus, even if we accepted that relentless economic growth were predictable and that this correlated reliably with well-being, we would have no reason to believe that all members of future generations will be better off than we are. Indeed, we should expect the opposite. Setting aside wishful thinking, we should expect that some members of future generations will be worse off than we are.[34] Thus, pure discounting in an effort to prevent the less well off (us) from bearing the burden of sacrificing for the better off (them) will misfire in relation to at least some members of future generations.

The last argument on behalf of pure discounting that we will consider is an argument from excessive sacrifice. By making sacrifices, we can give future generations a better world and a better life. But, if we give the interests of future generations fully equal consideration and consider effects of present sacrifices far into the future, it may seem that we must make very extensive sacrifices to squeeze out maximal future (and overall) benefit. This approach is unfair in its demands of us. To protect against an expectation of excessive sacrifice, we should discount future well-being.

This argument makes the good point that there are limits to the sacrifices we should be expected to make for the sake of future generations. But it does not really justify pure discounting. Rather, it recommends acceptance of a principle of fair equality among generations, according to which *no* generation should be expected to make sacrifices beyond some amount.[35] This would represent a departure from classical utilitarianism, which would endorse whatever arrangement would maximize expected well-being even if that arrangement demanded extreme sacrifices from some generation. Yet it is consistent with the general idea of equal consideration, which can take a wide variety of specific forms including, as here, human rights that include a right not to be required to undergo certain kinds or degrees of sacrifice. A principle of fair equality among generations is therefore compatible with the thesis that we should reject pure discounting.

In conclusion, we should not discount the well-being of future generations. What matters most, from the standpoint of individual lifestyle choices and public policy, is that we take the interests of future people seriously, try not to cause great harm, and conduct ourselves as good stewards of our environment, economy, gene pool, species, and so forth. Fortunately, there is no need to be extremely precise about predicted consequences in the very long-term future. Nor should we consider making enormous sacrifices that would make us very poorly off. We have enough information to know that modest sacrifices now in the way of energy consumption can make a huge difference in preventing disastrous climate change, and that we should make such changes. In the United States, we will surely have to make some changes in our tax policies (fewer tax breaks for rich individuals, oil companies, and other undeserving beneficiaries; perhaps somewhat higher taxes for all tax payers) and in Social Security and Medicare to preserve reasonable fiscal health for the next few generations. What we must not do is act in a way that leaves a much worse world for future generations on the assumption that their interests are not very important.

So far, then, in this chapter, it has been argued that future people will have full moral status, that the ways in which our actions predictably affect them is a matter of justice, and that their interests should not be discounted. But what if irresponsible action today will predictably leave future individuals a less good world than we could and should have left them—but the individuals who come into existence would not have existed had we acted more responsibly? Surely irresponsible choices today are subject to moral criticism, but if future persons are no worse off for them, how are we to understand the wrongdoing involved? We return to the nonidentity problem.

NONIDENTITY AGAIN: HOW TO EXPLAIN THE WRONG OF IRRESPONSIBLE CHOICES THAT LEAVE A WORSE WORLD FOR POSTERITY?

Gregory Kavka asks us to imagine

a society choosing between heavy investment in either solar energy systems or nuclear fission power plants in order to meet its projected energy needs

over the next few generations. Monetary investment costs per unit of out-
put will be slightly lower if the nuclear option is pursued. However, there is
no storage or disposal system for nuclear wastes that is expected to contain
them safely for more than a few generations. Hence, if the nuclear plan is
pursued, there would very likely be radioactive leakage that would cause
the deaths of thousands of people in future generations.[36]

It would surely be irresponsible to pursue the nuclear option considering its
expected cost of thousands of premature deaths and the fact that the safer
option would be only slightly more expensive to the current generation.

But explaining the nature of the wrong involved in this choice proves difficult due to the facts of nonidentity. Suppose the unsafe nuclear plant is built
and 200 years later thousands of people are dying from illnesses caused by the
predictable radioactive leakage. Suppose also that their lives, on the whole, are
worth living despite their illnesses and premature deaths—also (somewhat
unrealistically) that at the time of choosing the nuclear option it was predictable that radioactive leakage would not make the affected lives not worth living.
Now consider the effects of the policy choice on the identities of later people.
Building the nuclear power plant rather than taking the more responsible
course of building solar energy systems entailed that certain jobs would be created, that particular supplies would be needed at the job sites, that some of
businesses in the vicinity of the new jobs would have more customers, and so
on. These relatively direct effects of the nuclear option in turn affected where
new workers would live, where they would go, and who would meet whom. The
latter, of course, affected who would reproduce with whom, which in turn
determined who later comes into the world. After 200 years of causal ripple
effects of the initial policy choice—nuclear power rather than solar energy—it
seems likely to be true of everyone who comes into being that she would not
have existed had the alternative policy option been selected. Now consider
Roberto, a victim of exposure to nuclear radiation. Roberto is dying of illnesses
caused by this exposure, yet his life has been worth living. Was he harmed by
the irresponsible selection of the nuclear option? Not if harm involves being
made worse off, because he would not have existed had the other major option
been selected. Was Roberto wronged? There is reason to think not since he
should prefer having a worthwhile, if compromised, life to having no life at all.
If he was not wronged, is there a way to vindicate the intuition that selection of
the nuclear option was irresponsible and wrong? These and related questions
constitute the nonidentity problem as it applies to future generations.[37]

In Chapter 6, we examined the nonidentity problem as it applies to procreative choices. There we examined a wide variety of proposed solutions. Having
done so, we will be briefer in this discussion of the nonidentity problem. But we

will not simply refer back to Chapter 6 because here we encounter the problem in a different context: decisions that affect the condition of the world that we leave for future generations.

One option is to deny—contrary to what we are assuming at this stage of our discussion—that we have any obligations to, or even regarding, future generations. In one of the pioneering discussions of the nonidentity problem, Thomas Schwartz asserted that "[w]hatever we may owe ourselves or our near posterity, *we've no obligation extending indefinitely or even terribly far into the future to provide any widespread, continuing benefits to our descendants*."[38] His reasoning is simple: Whatever policy we choose will be numerical-identity-affecting, so we can neither benefit nor harm those who come into being, since they would not have existed had we taken another choice. Crucial to his reasoning is the person-affecting intuition: that an action is wrong only if it wrongs someone.[39]

Most commentators have rejected Schwartz's approach, maintaining that we do have obligations to future generations (and not only those closest in time to us). These thinkers would agree that selecting the nuclear option in our thought-experiment is morally wrong. The task, of course, is to explain how it can be wrong despite the fact of nonidentity.

There have been several attempts from within the contract tradition to address the nonidentity problem as it relates to future generations. Although Rawls is credited with providing the first systematic account of obligations to future generations—an account that proposes a "just savings" principle to govern what each generation ought to save for the next generation[40]—he was unaware of the nonidentity problem and did not address it. Nor does his theory seem capable of handling this problem. The imaginary contractors featured in the original position, although stripped of knowledge of their particular circumstances and other bias-inviting information regarding themselves, *do* know that they will be born into one generation or another. But such certainty of future existence is precisely what is lacking in nonidentity cases, so the principles of justice on which contractors would agree hold no promise of illuminating the nonidentity problem.[41]

Fully aware of the nonidentity problem, Joseph Mazor addresses it from the perspective of what he calls "liberal theories of justice."[42] This perspective, as he understands it, is closely related to the classical contract tradition in that both embrace a largely Humean view of the "circumstances of justice," from which it follows that we do not stand in relations of justice to future people. So Mazor concedes that present people do not have justice-based obligations to future people to conserve natural resources. But he argues that "present people can (and do) have obligations *to each other* to conserve natural resources *for* future people."[43] His argument exploits the idea that contemporaries can have obligations to each other regarding resource allocation for persons who will come into existence while they, the contemporaries, are still alive; and argues on behalf of more distant future generations by showing how the case of two over-lapping generations can be reiterated like links of a chain leading to persons in the more distant future.

Although ingenious, Mazor's response to the nonidentity problem has sev-eral disadvantages. First, it accepts the Hume-Rawls doctrine of the circum-stances of justice, which we criticized earlier, and the individual-affecting intuition—which holds that any wrong action must wrong at least one indi-vidual—an intuition we rejected in Chapter 6. Now, Mazor could reply that accepting the doctrine of the circumstances of justice along with the individ-ual-affecting intuition simply makes his task more challenging; more power to his approach, if it succeeds, for meeting this challenge. Fair enough, but I do not think his approach is satisfactory. *For it mislocates the wrong in irresponsible choices that affect future generations.* On Mazor's view, we wrong only *other presently living people* when we make irresponsible choices that negatively affect future generations. But, as discussed in Chapter 6, it seems that much of the wrong in such choices involves a kind of harming—which we eventually ana-lyzed as victimless harming—a kind of damage that is done in the future.[44]

Earlier in this chapter, we saw that Scanlon's contract theory has certain ad-vantages over theories that embrace the classical view of the circumstances of justice. Does Scanlon's view offer a viable solution to the nonidentity problem as it concerns future generations? The answer, I think, is yes and no. Yes, insofar as Scanlon's view could condemn irresponsible choices such as the selection of the nuclear option insofar as any principle that would allow such a choice is a principle that future people could reasonably reject. On the other hand, Scan-lon's view is limited to the portion of morality that involves *what people owe each other* and, as we saw in Chapter 6, the harm in nonidentity cases, which is literally victimless, can only be captured in impersonal consequentialist terms. Scanlon's view, although admirable, is radically incomplete as an account of morality because it excludes a portion of morality that must be invoked in a full and adequate response to the nonidentity problem.

We therefore return to the solution defended in Chapter 6: *Embrace a hybrid ethical theory with both individual-affecting and impersonal components.* The idea, again, is to think of beneficence and nonmaleficence in individual-affecting terms when such terms apply—that is, when our actions make particular indi-viduals better or worse off. But in cases of nonidentity such as the case intro-duced at the beginning of this section, we should think in the impersonal terms of making the world better or worse than it otherwise might be, depending on what action we take. In these cases, which include those involving future gen-erations beyond some relatively small expanse of time (that is, once the fact of nonidentity is established), we may invoke the concept of *victimless harm*: the bringing about of states of affairs that are worse than one could and should bring about, even though no individual is made worse off. The imposition of victimless harm is a central part of the wrong that is committed in the selection of the nuclear option rather than the safer, slightly more expensive option of solar power.

But the wrong in this and other nonidentity cases involving future genera-tions has other components as well. First, in most if not all cases of this kind, those who made the irresponsible decision that led to impersonal harm showed *insufficient regard and respect* for future generations. They did not take the irre-sponsible decision, fully aware of the fact of nonidentity, just so that certain individuals would come into existence with worthwhile lives. No, the decision-makers displayed an uncaring attitude towards any and all future people who might come into being—and, in this way, committed a virtue-based moral of-fense that can be understood in individual-affecting terms. In this respect, those who came into being *were* wronged, although not harmed, by the irre-sponsible choice made long before their births.

Additionally, as noted earlier, the irresponsible choice surely violated princi-ples that future people could not reasonably reject and therefore had compelling reason to accept, the focus of Scanlon's approach. Whatever the precise content of such principles, they would require taking appropriate account of the interests of those who would inherit the world and would accordingly demand some degree of sacrifice on the part of present people in the name of responsible stew-ardship of resources, prevention of later harm (whether individual-affecting or victimless), and so on; there is no need for such principles to be individual-affecting in their formulation. And the modest additional expenditure required by the option of solar energy would have been within the range of sacrifice required by the relevant principles. The same is true of rules that would be justi-fied within the more viable forms of rule-consequentialism: They need not be individual-affecting (indeed, their formulation would blur the distinction between individual-affecting and impersonal considerations), they would require responsible stewardship, and the choice made in the case under consideration would violate them. In this interesting way, the individual-affecting approach of "what we owe to each other" and the impersonal approach of consequentialism can find common cause in addressing the nonidentity problem as it applies to future generations.

We do have obligations to future generations. Insofar as they are grounded in the moral importance of avoiding victimless harm, they are obligations to future generations considered, impersonally, as a collective. Insofar as they are grounded in the moral importance of showing, through our choices, sufficient regard and respect for people, they are obligations to future persons considered as particular individuals. Insofar as they are grounded in obligations to act in accordance with principles and rules that people could not reasonably reject, or that are most conducive to good consequences in the long run, our obligations to future generations are both impersonal and personal.

NOTES

1. The first five paragraphs of this chapter borrow significantly from the editors' introduction to chap. 10 in Thomas Mappes, Jane Zembaty, and David De-Grazia (eds.), *Social Ethics*, 8th edition (New York: McGraw-Hill, 2012), pp. 517–19.

2. See Intergovernmental Panel on Climate Change, *Climate Change 2007: The Physical Science Basis* (Cambridge: Cambridge University Press, 2007); National Academy of Sciences, *Climate Change Science: An Analysis of Some Key Questions* (Washington, DC: National Academies Press, 2001); American Meteorological Society, *Bulletin of the American Meteorological Society* 84 (2003): 508; American Geophysical Union, *Eos* 84 (51) (2003): 574; and American Association for the Advancement of Science (http://www.ourplanet.com/aaas/pages/atmos02.html). For a summary of these findings (except that she cites an earlier IPCC report than the one cited above), see Naomi Oreskes, "The Scientific Consensus on Climate Change," *Science* 306 (December 3, 2004): 1686.

3. See D.S. Arndt, M.O. Baringer, and M.R. Johnson (eds.), *State of the Climate in 2009*, published as a special supplement in *Bulletin of the American Meteorological Society* 91 (7) (2010): S1–S224 and "The Truth about Global Warming: More Evidence from Respected Sources" (editorial), *The Washington Post* (August 2, 2010), p. A12.

4. Possibilities for grounding the stewardship obligations, which do not straightforwardly fall under the rubric of nonmaleficence, include these: (1) ground them in nonmaleficence by defending a relatively broad conception of harm; (2) ground them in the Lockean proviso that, when appropriating public resources for private ownership and use, one must leave "as much and as good" for others to use (see John Locke, *Second Treatise of Government* [1690], Chapter V, "Of Property"); and (3) ground them in obligations to benefit those in need. Thanks to Jeff Brand-Ballard for a thought-provoking discussion of these possibilities.

5. Justice between generations includes not only possible obligations to future generations, the topic of this chapter, but also possible obligations to past generations or particular individuals from the past. For an overview, see Lukas Meyer, "Intergenerational Justice," *Stanford Encyclopedia of Philosophy* (http://plato.stanford.edu/entries/justice-intergenerational/; first published April 2003, revised February 2008).

6. Henry Sidgwick, *The Methods of Ethics* (1874), p. 385. This historical note appears in Peter Laslett and James Fishkin, "Introduction: Processional Justice," in Laslett and Fishkin (eds.), *Justice between Age Groups and Generations* (New Haven: Yale University Press, 1992), p. 19.

7. John Rawls, *A Theory of Justice* (Cambridge, MA: Harvard University Press, 1971), sect. 44.

8. Derek Parfit, *Reasons and Persons* (Oxford: Clarendon, 1984), Part IV.

9. Some authors advance a similar argument about rights—that one can have rights only if one exists, as future individuals do not—without considering the intermediary condition of having interests. See, e.g., Wilfred Beckerman and Joanna Pasek, *Justice, Posterity, and the Environment* (New York: Oxford University Press, 2001), pp. 15–20 and Richard de George, "The Environment, Rights, and Future Generations," in Earnest Partridge (ed.), *Responsibilities to Future Generations* (New York: Prometheus, 1981), p. 161. My reply to this reasoning and parts of the remaining discussion in this section draw substantially from my "Just(ice) in Time for Future Generations: A Response to Hockett and Herstein," *George Washington Law Review* 77 (2009), pp. 1223–6.

10. See Albert Einstein, *Relativity*, trans. Robert Lawson (New York: Henry Holt, 1921).

11. Cf. Jan Narveson, "Future People and Us," in R. I. Sikora and Brian Barry (eds.), *Obligations to Future Generations* (Philadelphia: Temple University Press, 1978), p. 39.

12. For a helpful introduction to some of the theoretical possibilities, see Brian Greene, *The Fabric of the Cosmos* (New York: Vintage, 2004).

13. Here I find common cause with Joel Feinberg, "The Rights of Animals and Unborn Generations," in Joel Feinberg, *Rights, Justice, and the Bounds of Liberty* (Princeton: Princeton University Press, 1981), pp. 181–2 and Meyer, "Intergenerational Justice," sect. 2.1.

14. See, e.g., Ori Herstein, "The Identity and (Legal) Rights of Future Generations," *George Washington Law Review* 77 (2009), pp. 1181–82.

15. But I reject any *general* principle of correlativity between rights and obligations, which would include obligations that are not directed to particular individuals. For one thing, we have obligations of beneficence—for example, to contribute appropriately to charities—that do not correlate with anyone's rights. Moreover, due to the fact of nonidentity (as discussed later), our obligations to future generations may not always correlate with rights.

16. Roughly this reasoning appears in Beckerman and Pasek, *Justice, Posterity, and the Environment*, p. 16.

17. See John Stuart Mill, *Utilitarianism* (1863), chap. 5 and Rawls, *A Theory of Justice*.

18. Brian Barry, "Circumstances of Justice and Future Generations," in Sikora and Barry, *Obligations to Future Generations*, p. 205.

19. Lukas, "Intergenerational Justice," sect. 1. Drawing from David Hume's reflections on justice, Rawls summarizes the circumstances of justice as involving rough equality (requiring reciprocity and a balance of power), moderate scarcity of resources, and moderate selfishness among moral agents (*Theory of Justice*, pp. 126–7). In our discussion, we may assume that moderate scarcity and moderate selfishness obtain, so we need not discuss these factors. For an excellent analysis and critique of the Hume-Rawls view, see Barry, "Circumstances of Justice and Future Generations."

20. I emphasize *material* benefit to note a contrast with such other alleged benefits as an enhanced reputation or demonstrations of respect, which some thinkers believe presently existing individuals can confer on earlier generations or individuals.

21. See Thomas Hobbes, *Leviathan* (1651); Locke, *Second Treatise of Civil Government*; Rawls, *A Theory of Justice*; and T. M. Scanlon, *What We Owe to Each Other* (Cambridge, MA: Harvard University Press, 1998).

22. The classical source is Hobbes, *Leviathan*. A prominent contemporary representative is David Gautier, *Morals by Agreement* (Oxford: Oxford University Press, 1986).

23. *A Theory of Justice*, p. 127.

24. Barry develops both of these examples ("Circumstances of Justice and Future Generations," pp. 221–22).

25. For good discussions, see Allen Buchanan, "Justice as Reciprocity Versus Subject-Centered Justice," *Philosophy and Public Affairs* 19 (1990): 227–52 and Martha Nussbaum, *Frontiers of Justice* (Cambridge, MA: Harvard University Press, 2006), chap. 2.

26. I owe this observation to Barry, "Circumstances of Justice and Future Generations," pp. 229–33.

27. *Theory of Justice*, chap. 3.

28. *What We Owe to Each Other*, p. 185.

29. Elizabeth Ashford and Tim Mulgan, "Contractualism," *Stanford Encyclopedia of Philosophy* (http://plato.stanford.edu/entries/contractualism/; first published August 30, 2007), sect. 9.

30. See John Broome, "Discounting the Future," *Philosophy and Public Affairs* 23 (1994), pp. 129–31.

31. Cf. Tyler Cowen and Derek Parfit, "Against the Social Discount Rate," in Laslett and Fishkin, *Justice Between Age Groups and Generations*, p. 150.

32. See, e.g., Beckerman and Pasek, *Justice, Posterity, and the Environment*, chap. 6.

33. See, e.g., David Myers and Ed Diener, "The Pursuit of Happiness," *Scientific American* (May 1996): 70–72.

34. Cowen and Parfit, "Against the Social Discount Rate," p. 148.

35. See ibid, p. 149.

36. Gregory Kavka, "The Paradox of Future Individuals," *Philosophy and Public Affairs* 11 (1982), p. 97. The question of nuclear safety is much in the public's consciousness at the time of this writing because a recent tsunami has caused several nuclear plants in Japan to leak radioactive material into the environment.

37. Some of the earliest works to recognize this problem are Derek Parfit, "On Doing the Best for Our Children," in Michael Bayles (ed.) *Ethics and Population* (Cambridge, MA: Schenkman, 1976), pp. 100–102; Robert Adams, "Existence, Self-Interest, and the Problem of Evil," *Nous* 13 (1979), p. 57; Thomas Schwartz, "Obligations to Posterity," in Sikora and Barry, *Obligations to Future Generations* 3–13; and Kavka, "The Paradox of Future Generations."

38. "Obligations to Posterity," p. 3.

39. Ibid, pp. 11–12.
40. *A Theory of Justice*, sect. 44.
41. Jeffrey Reiman neglects this point in addressing the nonidentity problem from a Rawlsian perspective ("Being Fair to Future People: The Nonidentity Problem in the Original Position," *Philosophy and Public Affairs* 35 [2007]: 69–92).
42. Joseph Mazor, "Liberal Justice, Future People, and Natural Resource Conservation," *Philosophy and Public Affairs* 38 (2010): 380–408.
43. Ibid, p. 384.
44. Further, although we cannot enter into details here, Mazor's argument that we wrong our contemporaries with such choices requires a strong assumption about rights to equal resources and is hardly immune to challenge.

INDEX